Mediastinal Tumors
Update 1995

Contributors

M.S. Allen · J.D. Bitran · L. Delbridge · B. De Vries · L.P. Faber
R.J. Ginsberg · T.W. Griffin · R.F. Heitmiller · S. Keshavjee
W.-J. Koh · J. LeBlanc · R.B. Lee · P.J. Loehrer, Sr.
W.J. Marasco · D.J. Mathisen J.I. Miller, Jr. · S.H. Petersdorf
T.S. Reeve · M. Roach III · J. Somers · C.R. Thomas, Jr.
S. Vijayakumar · J.C. Wain · E.W. Wilkins, Jr. · D.E. Wood
C.D. Wright

Edited by

Douglas E. Wood and Charles R. Thomas, Jr.

Foreword by

Luther W. Brady and Hans-Peter Heilmann

With 55 Figures and 21 Tables

Springer-Verlag

Berlin Heidelberg New York
London Paris Tokyo
Hong Kong Barcelona
Budapest

Douglas E. Wood, MD
Head, Section of General Thoracic Surgery
Division of Cardio-thoracic Surgery
Department of Surgery, SA-25
University of Washington
1959 NE Pacific Street
Seattle, WA 98195
USA

Charles R. Thomas, Jr., MD
Fellow, Department of Radiation Oncology, RC-08
Former Assistant Professor, Division of Oncology
Department of Medicine
University of Washington
1959 NE Pacific Street
Seattle, WA 98195
USA

MEDICAL RADIOLOGY · Diagnostic Imaging and Radiation Oncology

Continuation of
Handbuch der medizinischen Radiologie
Encyclopedia of Medical Radiology

ISBN 3-540-58750-0 Springer-Verlag Berlin Heidelberg New York

CIP data applied for

Typesetting: Macmillan India Ltd., Bangalore 25

SPIN: 10487521   21/3130/SPS – 5 4 3 2 1 0 – Printed on acid-free paper

Foreword

Primary mediastinal tumors are relatively rare. The relative incidence of these tumors indicates that neurogenic tumors are the most common tumor seen constituting 21% of all cases, thymomas 19%, lymphomas 12.5%, germ cell tumors 10%, primary carcinomas 4.6%, mesenchymal tumors 6%, endocrine tumors 6%, cysts 18%. In adults, the majority of thyroid tumors, thymomas, mediastinal germ cell tumors and teratomas are located in the superior and anterior mediastinum. Of the neurogenic tumors 18% are located in the posterior mediastinum, and 50% of mediastinal lymphomas are in the middle mediastinum. In adults, the incidence of anterosuperior, middle and posterior mediastinal tumors is about 54%, 20% and 26% respectively. However, in children the posterior mediastinum contains 63% of the lesions, the anterior mediastinum contains 26% and the middle mediastinum 11%. The majority of the tumors are benign in character with a ratio of benign to malignant of about 60 to 40. The relative incidence of malignant mediastinal tumors in children is about 50%.

Even though mediastinal tumors are not common, they represent a unique problem with regards to treatment whether by surgery, radiation therapy and/or systemically administered chemotherapy.

The volume by WOOD and THOMAS deals with each of these issues in detail and presents a logical and important approach to the management of mediastinal tumors.

Philadelphia
Hamburg
January 1995

LUTHER W. BRADY
HANS-PETER HEILMANN

Preface

Mediastinal tumors present a fascinating and varied array of benign and malignant neoplasms. Cardiothoracic surgeons, general surgeons, medical and radiation oncologists, radiologists, pulmonologists, pediatricians, endocrinologists, and pathologists are all involved in the diagnosis and management of mediastinal tumors. Due to this wide spectrum of diseases and specialists, the literature on mediastinal tumors is scattered through the journals of multiple disciplines. As a result, many physicians do not have a clear understanding of this diverse array of tumors. In the past few years diagnostic techniques have improved with serum tumor markers. MRI, and more sophisticated imaging by CT and ultrasound. At the same time, advances in chemotherapy, radiation, and surgery have improved the outcomes for tumors that were previously "incurable" and interdisciplinary cooperation has resulted in many multimodality treatment protocols. This volume is aimed at consolidating the literature and providing a concise guide and reference to the state-of-the-art diagnosis and management of mediastinal tumors. We have enlisted thoracic surgeons, medical and radiation oncologists, and radiologists who are experienced in specific mediastinal tumors to provide thorough updates in their area of expertise. We greatly appreciate their important contributions to the field and to this supplement.

Seattle, WA 98195, USA
February 1995

DOUGLAS E. WOOD
CHARLES R. THOMAS, Jr.

Acknowledgement. We wish to give our sincere thanks to TERRI BODENMAN for all her help and hard work in preparing this volume. Without her dedication and perseverance this issue would probably be titled *Mediastinal Tumors: Update 1997.*

Contents

1 Diagnosis of Mediastinal Masses

JOHANNE LEBLANC and DOUGLAS E. WOOD

CONTENTS

1.1 Introduction

The mediastinum is defined as the space between the two pleural cavities extending from the thoracic inlet to the diaphragm. It is bounded by the sternum anteriorly and the vertebral bodies posteriorly. The paravertebral gutters have traditionally been included when considering mediastinal masses.

The mediastinum can be divided into three or four compartments and a variety of definitions have been used, adding confusion to the radiologic and surgical literature. The most commonly used definition divides the mediastinum into anterior, middle, and posterior compartments. The anterior mediastinum is bounded anteriorly by the sternum and posteriorly by the pericardium, brachiocephalic vessels, and aorta. It contains the thymus gland, internal mammary vessels, and lymph nodes. The middle mediastinum is bounded anteriorly and

JOHANNE LEBLANC, M.D., Clinical Assistant Professor, University of Washington, Department of Radiology, Group Health Cooperative of Puget Sound, 215, 15th Ave., Seattle, WA 98102, USA
DOUGLAS E. WOOD, M.D., Head, Section of General Thoracic Surgery, Assistant Professor, Division of Cardiothoracic Surgery, SA-25, University of Washington, Seattle, WA 98195, USA

posteriorly by the pericardium and great vessels. It contains the pericardium and the heart, the ascending and transverse aorta, the brachiocephalic vessels, the pulmonary artery and veins, the inferior and superior vena cavae, and the trachea and main bronchi with their contiguous lymph nodes. The posterior mediastinum is bounded anteriorly by the pericardium and posteriorly by the chest wall including the paravertebral gutters. It includes the esophagus, azygos and hemi-azygos veins, nerves, fat and lymph nodes [1].

Malignant mediastinal lymph nodes may be primary or secondary in origin. Mediastinal metastatic neoplasms usually arise from lymphatic spread from lung, esophageal, breast, thyroid, or gastric primaries to mediastinal lymph nodes. We will devote our discussion to primary tumors of the mediastinum, and in this chapter will present the fundamentals of the workup and diagnosis of mediastinal masses. Subsequent chapters written by experienced radiologists, oncologists, and thoracic surgeons will specifically outline the presentation and management of the wide variety of mediastinal neoplasms.

1.2 General Diagnostic Features

The incidence and location of primary mediastinal tumors in children is clearly different than in adults. Collected series have shown that neurogenic tumors and foregut cysts are nearly twice as common in children with mediastinal masses than in adults and in children make up 39% and 18% of the mediastinal masses respectively. Germ cell tumors and lymphomas each contribute about 13% in both children and adults. Thymomas make up 21% of adult mediastinal masses but are quite uncommon in children. Miscellaneous tumors and cysts produce the other 20% in children and adults [2]. Approximately two-thirds of mediastinal tumors are symptomatic in children while only one-third produce symptoms in adults [3]. Asymptomatic neoplasms are usually found during routine chest radiographs. Signs and symptoms that do occur result from invasion or compression of local structures, the presence of infection, or the release of endocrine products.

Respiratory symptoms often predominate, particularly in infants and children, due to compression of the airway. Involvement of the esophagus may produce dysphagia or odynophagia. Anterior and middle mediastinal masses may produce superior vena cava syndrome and invasion into the chest wall usually produces pain. Pleural and pericardial effusions are possible and a chylothorax can occur from malignant lymphatic obstruction. Nerve involvement in the middle mediastinum may result in hoarseness or diaphragmatic paralysis, and in the posterior mediastinum may result in Horner's syndrome, upper extremity pain, back pain, or even paraplegia. Systemic signs of infection may lead to a diagnosis of an infected foregut cyst. Other systemic symptoms or signs may be present in both malignant and benign mediastinal tumors. These will be discussed separately in subsequent chapters.

The incidence of malignancy depends on the location of the mass, presence of symptoms and the age of the patient. Anterior mediastinal masses are more commonly malignant (59%) than are middle mediastinal masses (29%) or posterior mediastinal masses (16%) [4]. Asymptomatic patients with a mediastinal mass have a benign diagnosis 76% of the time while symptomatic patients have a malignant neoplasm 62% of the time [4]. The incidence of malignancy in mediastinal masses is greater in children than in adults. The most common mediastinal mass in children is a neurogenic tumor with an incidence of malignancy ranging from 60% to 85% [5,6], while the incidence of malignancy is only 1%–3% for neurogenic tumors in adults [7]. DAVIS and colleagues [8] found a lower incidence of malignancy in patients 10 years of age and younger, compared to the incidence of malignancy from the second to the fourth decades of life.

1.3 Diagnostic Studies

Mediastinal masses noted on chest radiograph can be narrowed down to a limited differential diagnosis based upon the patient's age, presence of symptoms, and location. All patients should undergo a thorough history and physical examination eliciting symptoms and signs of direct or indirect tumor invasion or involvement, as well as systemic signs of disease.

Routine laboratory studies will add little to the diagnosis of most mediastinal masses, but there are biochemical markers that should be obtained in certain clinical settings. All young men with an anterior mediastinal mass should have α-fetoprotein and β-HCG levels obtained to evaluate the presence of a nonseminomatous germ cell tumor. Infants and children with a paravertebral mass should have measurement of urinary catecholamines, metanephrines, and vanillylmandelic acid. Other markers have been useful for following the course of patients during treatment. Placental alkaline phosphatase has been used as a serum marker for patients with seminoma and neuron-specific enolase and chromograffin can be used as a marker for bronchial or thymic carcinoids [9].

1.4 Diagnostic Imaging of Mediastinal Masses in the Adult

Assessment of mediastinal abnormalities is a challenging task for the radiologist. The majority of these masses are found on conventional chest radiographs. With the advance of cross-sectional imaging, computed tomography (CT) has become the modality of choice to assess the specific characteristic of mediastinal masses or to detect them when an abnormality is clinically suspected. In selective cases, magnetic resonance imaging (MRI) is helpful due to its multiplanar possibilities to assess involvement of surrounding structures not answered by CT scan. It is especially useful for assessing vascular invasion or aneurysms, but also very useful in case of allergy to iodinated contrast agents. Ultrasonography is useful in some mediastinal masses, especially anterior masses, either to characterize a lesion as cystic or solid or to guide percutaneous biopsy. Radionuclide scanning plays an important role predominantly in the assessment of thyroid and parathyroid lesions.

Definition of the specific compartment in which the lesion is found and its radiologic characteristics are very helpful in narrowing down the differential diagnosis of the lesion involving the mediastinum.

1.4.1 Anterior Mediastinum

1.4.1.1 Thyroid

Substernal thyroid goiter is a common lesion arising from the cervical region in the superior and anterior mediastinum. It may even extend below the carina. Rarely, true ectopic thyroid tissue can be found in the mediastinum [10]. On plain film, it often presents as an asymptomatic paratracheal soft tissue mass that may contain calcifications and sometimes displaces the trachea laterally and occasionally anteriorly due to a retrotracheal component (Fig. 1.1).

Computed tomography provides excellent information in the assessment of the substernal goiter. Enlargement tends to arise from the inferior pole of a thyroid lobe and the mediastinal mass usually has a clear continuity with the often enlarged cervical thyroid. Substernal goiters have well-defined borders and often contain calcifications that are coarse or ring-like. They are heterogeneous, with areas of low density [11, 12]. Thyroid tissue is dense before contrast injection and enhanced after injection of iodinated contrast agent. The enlarged thyroid tends to insinuate into the mediastinum by displacing the great vessels laterally but sometimes

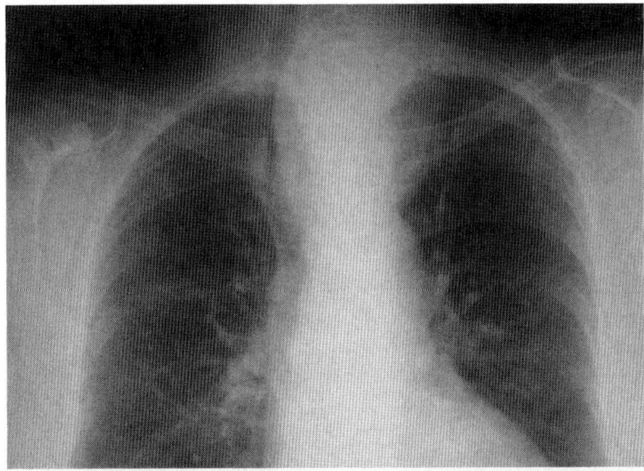

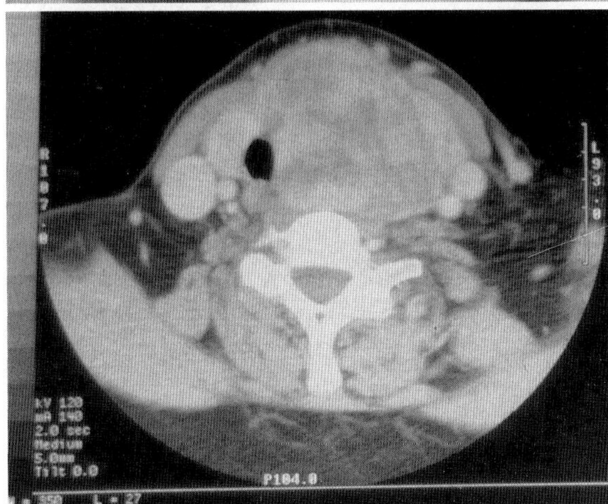

Fig. 1.1a, b. Intrathoracic goiter. **a** Chest radiograph demonstrating a large left paratracheal mass displacing the trachea to the right. **b** Enhanced CT scan showing a large heterogeneous mass with well-defined borders displacing the trachea to the right and the brachiocephalic vessels laterally

may encase the trachea, causing narrowing of the airway. Though other symptoms such as superior vena cava obstruction may occur, true superior vena cava syndrome is rare in the absence of malignancy [10].

Differentiating between benign and malignant lesions of the thyroid gland is usually not possible with imaging techniques. Irregular borders of the mass with or without invasion of the surrounding fat planes, presence of enlarged lymph nodes, and invasion of surrounding structures are all characteristics suggesting malignancy [13, 14]. MRI seldom adds additional information unless it is used to help determine vascular involvement.

Thyroid scintigraphy is extremely helpful and readily available to provide diagnostic information regarding an anterior mediastinal mass suspected to be an enlarged thyroid. In these cases, the nuclear scan will most often show an enlarged thyroid gland protruding in the upper mediastinum with multiple hot and cold nodules. It also has the advantage of providing information concerning the thyroid function.

1.4.1.2 Parathyroid

Four parathyroid glands are usually found in the cervical region. They can be supernumerary and ectopic. It is unusual to have a parathyroid adenoma presenting as a mediastinal mass. More commonly, patients will be diagnosed with primary hyperparathyroidism and a search made for the abnormal gland or glands.

Preoperative imaging in cases of primary hyperparathyroidism is often considered optional by the surgeon, but is mandatory in cases of persistent or recurrent hyperparathyroidism after cervical exploration. Ultrasound is considered the most valuable modality for the assessment of the cervical region. Real-time ultrasound will reveal the abnormal parathyroid as a small round well-defined hypoechoic mass.

Persistent hyperparathyroidism after surgery, however, is often due to an ectopic parathyroid gland. Eighty percent of ectopic parathyroids are located in the anterior mediastinum within or adjacent to the thymus at the level of the innominate vessels [10]. Ultrasound has a limited value when the ectopic lesion is in the mediastinum, where thallium-technetium subtraction scintigraphy and CT have proven useful. CT is performed with IV contrast and is most accurate with lesions measuring more than

1 cm. MRI is gaining acceptance and is also used successfully [15–17]. There is no well-established algorithm to determine which of these techniques is the best and in which order they should be used. It will depend mostly on the modality available and more than one technique is often required to confirm the diagnosis.

1.4.1.3 Thymus

The normal thymus gland fills the entire anterior mediastinum during infancy and at puberty starts to involute, completely disappearing in the adult. By age 25, the bilobed well-defined soft tissue density in the anterior mediastinum will usually be replaced by fat.

Thymoma is the most common mass of the anterior mediastinum in the adult [20] and is the most common thymic tumor. It may occur with a variety of systemic disorders, most frequently myasthenia gravis. Approximately 15% of patients with myasthenia gravis have a thymoma and approximately 35% of patients with thymoma have myasthenia gravis [1].

Roentgenographically, thymomas usually present as a soft tissue mass of the anterior mediastinum, sometimes asymmetric and projecting over a hilum. CT reveals a round, sometimes lobulated, well-defined soft tissue mass (Fig. 1.2). Calcification occurs in 7% and cysts may also be present [21]. Important characteristics suggestive of malignancy are evidence of vascular invasion, encasement, pericardial or cardiac invasion, or pleural metastases.

Magnetic resonance imaging of thymoma typically reveals a round or lobulated mass with a signal of intermediate intensity on T1-weighted images and increased intensity on T2-weighted images. Regions of high-intensity on T2-weighted images correspond to cystic or hemorrhagic areas [22, 23].

Despite the advance of imaging techniques, differentiation between benign and malignant thymoma remains impossible roentgenographically. Though loss of the surrounding fat planes, encasement of the surrounding structures, or detection of possible metastases are suggestive of malignancy, no precise radiologic criteria to determine malignancy are recognized. Diagnosis and staging should be determined in the operating room by the surgeon in conjunction with the pathologist [24].

Thymolipoma is a rare benign tumor. It is a soft tumor that may grow very large before it is recognized since it is usually asymptomatic. A thymolipoma may mimic an elevated hemidiaphragm or cardiomegaly since it can drape over the mediastinal structures or lay in one hemithorax. On CT a mass with fat density is identified that can contain discrete areas of soft tissue density representing small foci of thymic tissue and / or fibrous stroma. Because of its high fat content it will have a high signal intensity on T1-weighted images (Fig. 1.3).

Thymic cysts are benign lesions of the thymic gland. They can be found incidentally but also after radiation therapy to the mediastinum for Hodgkin's disease [25]. If a cyst exhibits low attenuation with CT numbers near water density, the diagnosis of a simple cyst can usually be made. Cysts will exhibit low signal intensity on T1-weighted images and high signal intensity on T2-weighted images on MR imaging.

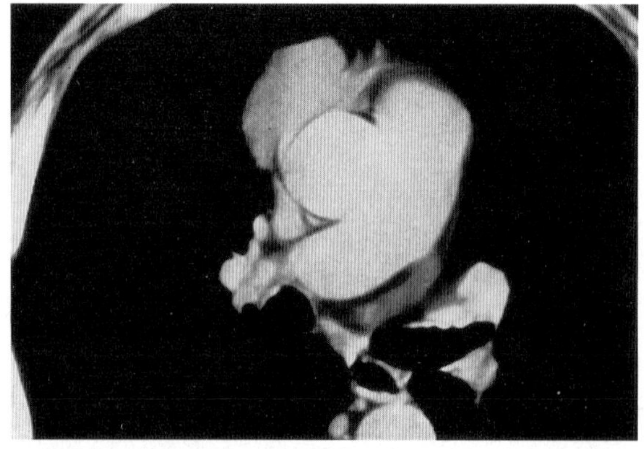

Fig. 1.2. Thymoma. Enhanced CT scan of the chest at the level of the right pulmonary artery showing a well-defined, homogeneous soft tissue mass, just anterior to the ascending aorta, in a patient with myasthenia gravis.

1.4.1.4 Germ Cell Tumors

Mediastinal germ cell neoplasms are tumors of the anterior mediastinum. Primary germ cell tumors include benign and malignant teratoma, seminoma, choriocarcinoma, and embryonal cell carcinoma. Malignant germ cell tumors are more common in males though benign tumors have no sex predilection.

The benign or mature teratoma represents the most common mediastinal germ cell tumor. These neoplasms are usually found in the adolescent and young adult. The roentgenologic diagnosis of benign teratoma is usually established by the demonstration of a smooth, round or oval mass that may contain a

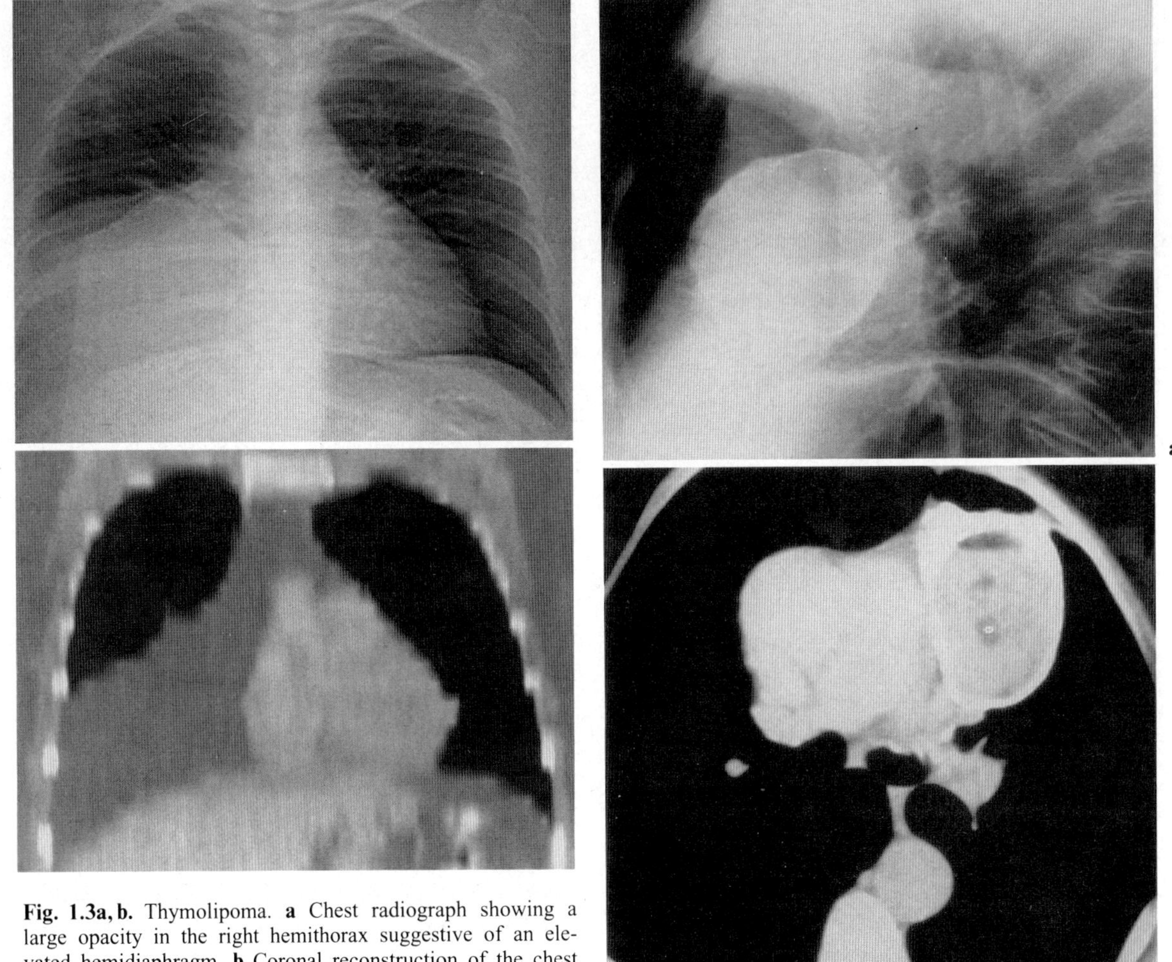

Fig. 1.3a, b. Thymolipoma. **a** Chest radiograph showing a large opacity in the right hemithorax suggestive of an elevated hemidiaphragm. **b** Coronal reconstruction of the chest CT showing the presence of a large fatty mass extending from the upper mediastinum to the right diaphragm, explaining the "pseudo-elevation" of the right hemidiaphragm

Fig. 1.4a, b. Benign teratoma. **a** Lateral chest radiograph showing a large partially calcified mass. **b** CT of the upper thorax demonstrating the large mass with calcified contour. The mass contains fat and a fat-fluid level

variable amount of fluid, fat, or calcification. A fat-fluid level can be seen in cystic teratomas (Fig 1.4). These lesions may be complicated by rapid increase in size due to bleeding. They can also rupture into the pleural space or pericardium [26, 27].

The most common type of malignant germ cell tumor is the seminoma. These are usually large soft tissue masses with smooth margins and can protrude on one or both sides of the mediastinum. They mostly have homogeneous attenuation. Seminomas may obliterate fat planes and calcification is characteristically absent [28] (Fig. 1.5). Nonseminomatous germ cell tumors may contain areas of low density representing cystic and/or necrotic changes. They have a tendency to have spiculated margins and fat planes are often obliterated [29, 30].

1.4.1.5 Lymphoma

Malignant lymphomas commonly cause anterior mediastinal node enlargement. The most common is Hodgkin's lymphoma of the nodular sclerosing type. HARMS and BROWN [13] reviewed the CT appearance of primary thoracic lymphoma in 95 patients and found that they most often present as a nonspecific solid anterior mediastinal mass that may contain areas of low density, felt to represent necrosis. These masses can be well-defined but may also exhibit infiltration of the surrounding lung parenchyma (Fig. 1.6). Eighty-six percent of these patients had lymph node enlargement elsewhere in the mediastinum. In addition, 15%–30% [1] of these

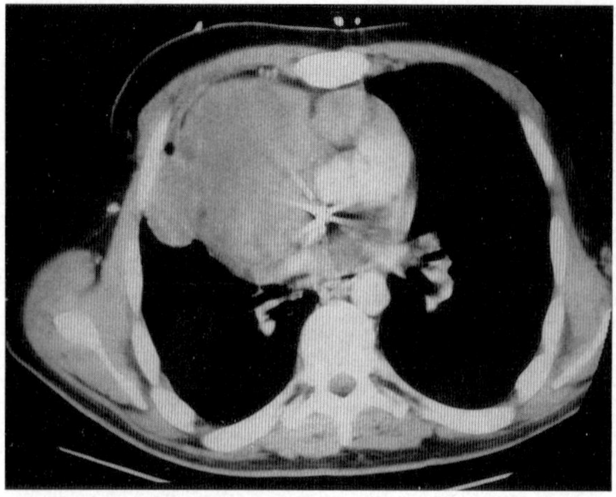

Fig. 1.5. Seminoma. Enhanced CT scan of the chest showing a large homogeneous right-sided soft tissue mass with well-defined borders displacing the mediastinum to the left

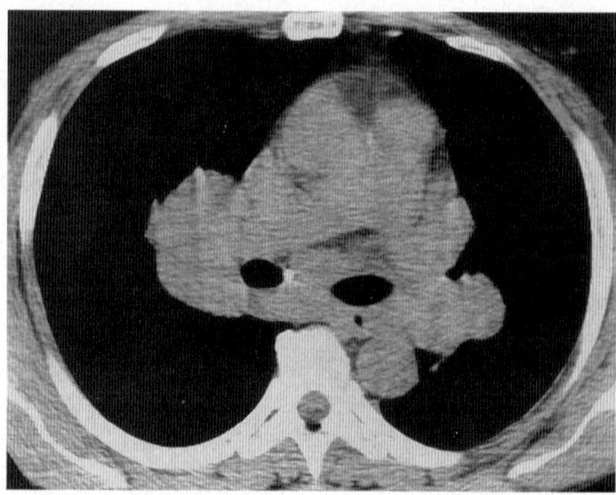

Fig. 1.7. Sarcoidosis. CT scan of the chest without contrast just below the carina, exhibiting markedly enlarged and symmetrically distributed hilar and mediastinal lymph nodes

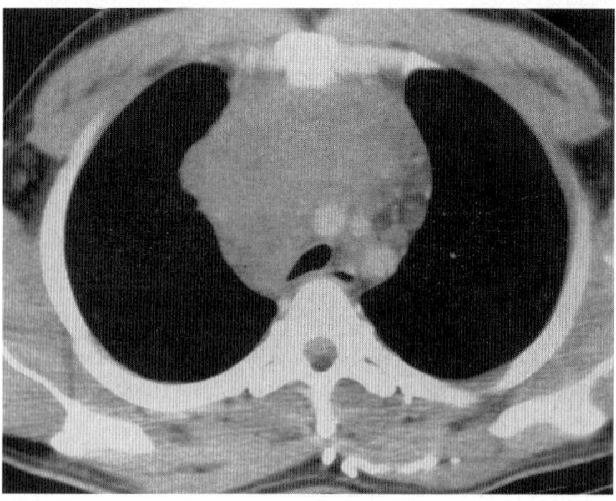

Fig. 1.6. Hodgkin's lymphoma. CT scan with contrast showing a large anterior mediastinal mass displacing the vessels posteriorly and compressing the trachea. Note the presence of collateral flow around the left scapula

patients have pleural effusions which are uncommon for other type of mediastinal masses.

1.4.2 Middle Mediastinum

1.4.2.1 Lymph Nodes

Enlargement of lymph nodes constitutes the most common middle mediastinal abnormality and most often reflects involvement by lymphomas, metastatic

carcinoma, granulomatous diseases, or infection (Fig. 1.7).

1.4.2.2 Primary Neoplasm of the Airway

Squamous cell carcinoma is the most common malignancy involving the trachea, representing approximately 50% of all tracheal neoplasms. Adenoid cystic carcinoma makes up 40%–45% of tracheal tumors and is often characterized by extensive local invasion. Many other rare neoplasms can involve the airway, such as chondromas, leiomyomas, neurofibromas, adenomas, granular cell tumors, carcinoid tumors, mucoepidermoid tumors, sarcomas, adenocarcinomas, and small cell carcinomas [31, 32].

On a standard roentgenogram, a tracheal neoplasm may be seen as an endoluminal soft tissue mass or a subtle thickening or irregularity of the tracheal wall. In the assessment of tracheal neoplasms, CT is the preferred method of evaluation for detecting mediastinal extension and local invasion (Fig. 1.8). Thin-section CT is helpful in the area of interest to assess both extension and endoluminal involvement and can be reconstructed in multiple planes. MRI is sometimes useful for assessment of the extension of the disease due to the multiplanar imaging capabilities. Conventional tomograms are still very important in the assessment of tracheal tumors and are especially important for surgical planning due to the good definition of longitudinal extent of disease and relationship to important anatomic landmarks.

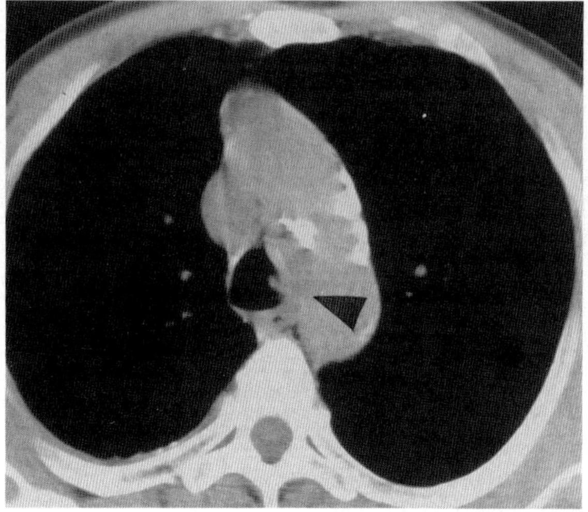

Fig. 1.8. Adenoid cystic carcinoma. Chest CT scan demonstrating a discrete soft tissue mass in the tracheal lumen arising from the left lateral tracheal wall

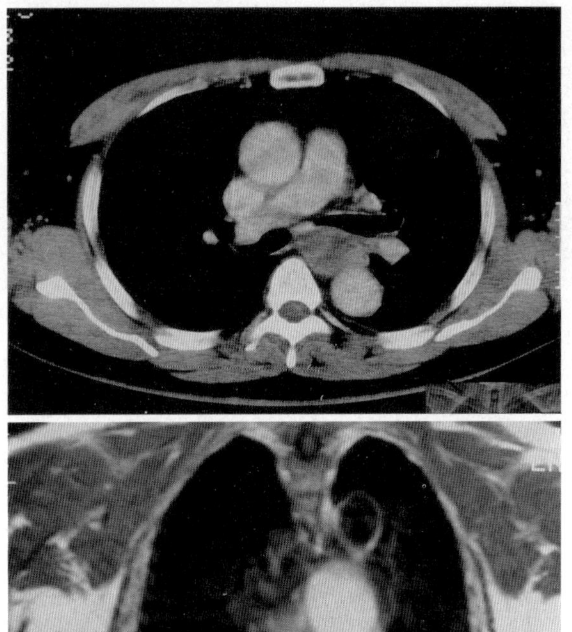

Fig. 1.9a, b. Bronchogenic cyst. **a** Chest CT showing a well-defined hypodense soft tissue mass in the left subcarinal region. **b** T1-weighted coronal image demonstrating a hyperintense mass. The bright signal is felt to be due to its hemorrhagic and/or proteinaceous content

1.4.2.3 Bronchogenic Cyst

Bronchogenic cysts are a congenital abnormality due to abnormal budding of the primitive tracheobronchial tree. They are well-defined soft tissue masses that can be intrapulmonary but most often are found in the mediastinum in the vicinity of the carina or the proximal tracheobronchial tree. An esophagogram may show smooth extrinsic compression on the esophagus. The CT appearance of bronchogenic cysts is well known. They present as well-defined masses. The CT numbers vary according to their content, which can be serous with CT numbers near water density, or proteinaceous and/or hemorrhagic with high CT numbers that would suggest a solid rather than a cystic mass [33]. Consequently appearance on MRI may range from that of a simple cyst with relatively low signal intensity on T1-weighted images and high signal on T2-weighted images to a high signal intensity on both T1- and T2-weighted images (Fig. 1.9) [34].

1.4.2.4 Pericardial Cyst

Pericardial cysts are benign mesothelial cysts. They are a well-defined soft tissue density usually located in the cardiophrenic angle. Though they usually have near water density on CT, there have been case reports of pericardial cysts with high CT numbers [35], probably due to mucoid or hemorrhagic

content. Thoracic ultrasound can be very useful, showing the characteristic ultrasound findings of a cyst.

1.4.2.5 Vascular Abnormalities

Significant dilatation of any arteries or veins in the mediastinum may suggest the presence of a mediastinal mass. Venous dilatation can be observed in cases of congenital abnormalities such as absence of the inferior vena cava with consequent dilatation of the azygos vein presenting with smooth widening of the right tracheobronchial angle. Venous dilatation also can be due to obstruction by a mediastinal mass such as enlarged lymph nodes or carcinoma or can even represent a normal variant.

Aneurysms of the aorta or great vessels as well as dilatation of the pulmonary arteries can present as middle mediastinal masses and can be assessed readily with enhanced CT scan or MRI.

1.4.3 Posterior Mediastinum

1.4.3.1 Neurogenic Tumors

Two predominant groups of neurogenic tumors are found in the posterior mediastinum. The neurofibroma, neurilemoma (schwannoma), and neurogenic sarcoma (malignant schwannoma) arise from the peripheral nerves. The second group, comprising the ganglioneuroma, ganglioneuroblastoma, and neuroblastoma, arise from the sympathetic ganglia.

Roentgenographically, their appearance is virtually identical. They are well-circumscribed paraspinal masses. The tumors arising from the sympathetic ganglia can contain calcifications. Bony erosions may occur in both groups but can be more subtle with ganglioneuroma [1]. The tumors originating from the peripheral nerves can have intraspinal involvement. When tumors abut the neural foramen, MRI is mandatory to evaluate the intraspinal extent of the lesion. Neurogenic tumors typically exhibit an intermediate signal on T1-weighted images and high signal on T2-weighted images. The use of gadolinium-DTPA is very useful in the assessment of the intradural extension [15].

1.4.3.2 Miscellaneous Posterior Mediastinal Masses

Diseases of the esophagus such as diverticulum, hiatus hernia, or neoplasm may present as a posterior mediastinal mass. When an esophageal pathology is suspected most often the investigation will start with an esophagogram. In most instances, if the abnormality represents a benign pathologic process this will be sufficient. In suspected neoplasms additional assessment with CT is extremely valuable for preoperative staging.

Diseases of the thoracic spine such as infectious spondylitis, primary or secondary neoplasms, and paravertebral hematomas due to trauma may cause paravertebral widening. Enlarged lymph nodes, meningocele and thoracic extramedullary hematopoiesis may present as a sharply defined paravertebral mass or masses.

1.5 Tissue Diagnosis and Staging

1.5.1 Needle Biopsy

Interventional radiology plays an important role in the investigation of these masses. It is simple, cost-effective and an alternative to more invasive diagnostic surgical procedures. Percutaneous biopsy using CT guidance is minimally invasive and has the advantage of giving access to all of the mediastinal compartments. Fluoroscopy and ultrasonography are also used as guiding imaging techniques but have more limitations [36, 37]. Percutaneous aspiration of bronchogenic cyst has been performed with success for both therapeutic and diagnostic purposes [38], though surgical excision remains the most accepted and recognized treatment for this type of lesion [34, 39].

1.5.2 Mediastinoscopy and Anterior Mediastinotomy

Mediastinoscopy was refined by CARLENS, who described and developed the mediastinoscope [40]. Mediastinoscopy allows exploration and biopsy of the paratracheal and tracheobronchial lymph nodes as well as masses along the trachea or its bifurcation. It is a simple and safe operative approach providing access to the middle mediastinum. In centers where this procedure is done frequently, morbidity requiring surgical treatment was found to occur only 0.3% of the time, with a total morbidity of 2% and no mortality [41, 42].

Anterior mediastinotomy, commonly known as the Chamberlain procedure, provides good access for direct biopsy of almost all lesions lying in the anterior mediastinum or the aortopulmonary window. Both right and left approaches through the second or third interspace or resecting costal cartilage give good access to the anterior mediastinum. A left anterior mediastinotomy allows easy and safe exposure to the aortopulmonary window and subaortic lymph nodes which are inaccessible during routine mediastinoscopy. Tumors can be directly biopsied during anterior mediastinotomy as well as assessed for extent and evidence of invasion as a preoperative staging procedure. A note of caution is emphasized, however, when biopsying tumors such as a thymoma which have a known potential for seeding viable tumor cells. For limited mediastinal masses that have a significant likelihood of being a thymoma, excision is often the diagnostic modality of choice to prevent the possibility of tumor seeding.

1.5.3 Thoracoscopy and Thoracotomy

Video-assisted thoracoscopy provides an excellent modality for examining most of the mediastinum.

It may be useful for biopsy of anterior, middle, and posterior mediastinal masses, and can be used to resect certain benign mediastinal cysts and tumors. The middle mediastinum below the level of the carina is inaccessible to mediastinoscopy or anterior mediastinotomy but is easily approached by video-assisted thoracoscopy. The disadvantages are that it requires violation of the pleural space and two-lung anesthesia, and it is currently seldom done as an outpatient procedure, as are mediastinoscopy and mediastinotomy. However, with rapid improvement in experience and equipment, thoracoscopy will likely play an increasing role in both the diagnosis and the management of mediastinal masses.

Median sternotomy or thoracotomy may be the only approach that is able to obtain tissue for diagnosis. In these cases the surgery is often diagnostic as well as therapeutic, with an excisional biopsy often acting as the definitive therapy.

1.6 Conclusion

The most important criteria for diagnosing mediastinal masses are age, symptoms, location, and radiographic characteristics. Most of the imaging strategy for mediastinal masses relies on the plain chest radiograph and CT scan. These techniques are extremely effective in identifying and delineating the lesion and in determining its location and tissue characteristics, and are consequently helpful in establishing a judicious differential diagnosis. If necessary, tissue diagnosis can be obtained by needle biopsy, limited surgical exploration, or surgical resection. Prognosis and treatment depend on the diagnosis and will be discussed in subsequent chapters.

References

1. Fraser RG, Pare JAP, Pare PD, Fraser RS, Genereux GP (1991) Diseases of the mediastinum. In: Fraser RG, Pare JAP, Pare PD, Fraser RS, Genereux GP (eds) Diagnosis of diseases of the chest, 3rd edn. Saunders, Philadelphia, pp 203–205
2. Shields TW (1991) Primary mediastinal tumors and cysts and their diagnostic investigation. In: Shields TW (ed) Mediastinal surgery. Lea & Febiger, Philadelphia, pp 111–117
3. Shields TW (1991) Lesions masquerading as primary mediastinal tumors or cysts. In: Shields TW (ed) Mediastinal surgery. Lea & Febiger, Philadelphia
4. Davis RD Jr, Oldham HN Jr, Sabiston DC Jr (1990) The mediastinum. In: Sabiston DC Jr, Spencer FC (eds) Surgery of the chest, vol I. Saunders, Philadelphia, pp 498–535
5. Reed JC, Hallet KK, Feigin DS (1978) Neural tumors of the thorax: subject review from the AFIP. Diagn Radiol 126: 9–17
6. Shields TW, Reynolds M (1988) Neurogenic tumors of the thorax. Surg Clin North Am 68: 645–668
7. Reed JC, Hallet KK, Feigin DS, Davidson KG, Walbaum PR, McCormack RJM (1978) Intrathoracic neural tumours. Thorax 33: 359–367
8. Davis PD Jr, Oldham HN Jr, Sabiston DC Jr (1987) Neoplasms of the mediastinum: recent changes in clinical presentation, methods of diagnosis, management, and results. Ann Thorac Surg 44: 229
9. Robinson PG, Radosevich JA (1991) Mediastinal tumor markers. In: Shields TW (ed) Mediastinal surgery. Lee & Febiger, Philadelphia, pp 62–76
10. Creswell LL, Wells SA Jr (1992) Mediastinal masses originating in the neck. Chest Surg North Am 2: 23–52
11. Bahist B, Ellis K, Gold RP (1983) Computed tomography of the intrathoracic goiters. Am J Roentgenol 140: 455–460
12. Glazer GM, Axel L, Moss AA (1982) CT diagnosis of mediastinal thyroid. Am J Roentgenol 138: 495–498
13. Pearlberg JL, Sandler MA, Talpos GB, Beurte GH (1989) Computed tomographic evaluation of thyroid disease. Comput Med Imaging Graph 13: 411–417
14. Silverman PM, Newman GE, Korobkin M, Workman JB, Moore AV, Coleman RE (1984) Computed tomography in the evaluation of thyroid disease. Am J Roentgenol 142: 897–902
15. Link KM, Samuels LJ, Loehr SP, Lesko NM (1993) MR imaging of the mediastinum. J Thorac Imaging 8: 34–53
16. Clark OH (1988) Mediastinal parathyroid tumors. Arch Surg 123: 1096–1099
17. Kang YS, Rosen K, Clark OH, Higgins CB (1993) Localization of abnormal parathyroid glands of the mediastinum with MR imaging. Radiology 189: 137–141
18. Naidich DP, Zerhouni EA, Siegelman SS (1991) In: Computed tomography and magnetic resonance of the thorax, 2nd edn. Raven Press, New York
19. Francis IR, Glazer GM, Bookstein FL, Gross BH (1985) The thymus re-examination of age related changes in size and shape. Am J Radiol 145: 249–254
20. Shields TW (1991) Thymic tumors. In: Shields TW (ed) Mediastinal surgery. Lea & Febiger, Philadelphia, pp 153–173
21. Brown LR, Aughenbaugh GL (1991) Masses of the anterior mediastinum: CT and MR imaging. Am J Roentgenol 157: 1171–1180
22. Sakai F, Sone S, Kiyono K, et al. (1992) MR imaging of thymoma: radiologic-pathologic correlation. Am J Roentgenol 158: 751–756
23. Molina PL, Siegel MJ, Glazer HS (1990) Thymic masses on MR imaging. Am J Roentgenol 155: 495–500
24. Wilkins EW, Grillo HC, Scannel JG, Moncure AC, Mathisen DJ (1991) Role of staging in prognosis and management of thymoma. Ann Thorac Surg 51: 888–892
25. Baron RL, Sagel SS, Baglan RJ (1981) Thymic cysts following radiation therapy for Hodgkins disease. Radiology 141: 593–597
26. Fulcher AS, Proto AV, Jolles H (1990) Cystic teratoma of the mediastinum: demonstration of fat-fluid level. Am J Roentgenol 154: 259–260
27. Yeoman LJ, Dalton HR, Adam EJ (1990) Fat-fluid level in pleural effusion as a complication of a mediastinal dermoid: CT characteristics. J Comput Assist Tomogr 14: 307
28. Polansky SM, Barwick KW, Ravin CE (1979) Primary mediastinal seminoma. Am J Roentgenol 132: 17–21

29. Lee KS, Im J-G, Han CH, Kim C-W, Kim WS (1989) Malignant germ cell tumors of the mediastinum: CT features. Am J Roentgenol 153: 947–951

30. Levitt RG, Husband JE, Glazer HS (1984) CT of primary germ-cell tumors of the mediastinum. Am J Roentgenol 142: 73–78

31. Naidich DP (1990) CT/MR correlation in the evaluation of tracheal neoplasia. Radiol Clin North Am 28: 555–571

32. Grillo HC, Mathisen DJ (1990) Primary tracheal tumors: treatment and results. Ann Thorac Surg 49: 69–77

33. Mendelson DS, Rose JS, Efremidis SC, Krischner PA, Cohen BA (1983) Bronchogenic cysts with high CT numbers. Am J Roentgenol 140: 463–465

34. Suen H, Mathisen DJ, Grillo HC, LeBlanc J, McLoud TC, Moncure AC, Hilgenberg AD (1993) Surgical management and radiological characteristics of bronchogenic cysts. Ann Thorac Surg 55: 476–481

35. Brunner DR, Whitley NO (1984) A pericardial cyst with high CT numbers. Am J Roentgenol 142: 279–280

36. Herman SJ, Holub RV, Weisbrod GL, Chamberlain DW (1991) Anterior mediastinal masses: utility of transthoracic needle biopsy. Radiology 180: 167–170

37. Wernecke K, Vassallo P, Peters PE, von Bassewitz DB (1989) Mediastinal tumors: biopsy under US guidance. Radiology 172: 473–476

38. Kuhlman JE, Fishman EK, Wang KP, Zerhouni EA, Siegelman SS (1988) Mediastinal cysts: diagnosis by CT and needle aspiration. Am J Roentgenol 150: 75–78

39. St-Georges R, Deslauriers J, Duranceau A et al. (1991) Clinical spectrum of bronchogenic cysts of the mediastinum and lung in the adult. Ann Thorac Surg 52: 6–13

40. Carlens E (1959) Mediastinoscopy: a method for inspection and tissue biopsy in the superior mediastinum. Chest 36: 343

41. Coughlin M, Deslauriers J, Beaulieu M, Fournier B, Piraux M, Rouleau J, Tardif A (1985) Role of mediastinoscopy in pretreatment staging in patients with primary lung cancer. Ann Thorac Surg 40: 556–560

42. Luke WP, Todd TRJ, Cooper JD (1986) Prospective of evaluation of mediastinoscopy for assessment of carcinoma of the lung. J Thorac Cardiovasc Surg 91: 53–56

2 Thymoma: Surgical Management

EARLE W. WILKINS, JR.

CONTENTS

2.1 Introduction

Although the term *thymoma* technically applies to any tumor arising within the thymus gland, it has come to mean a tumor of thymic epithelium only [1]. In their 1976 *Atlas of Tumor Pathology*, ROSAI and LEVINE [2] proposed "that the designation of thymoma be restricted to neoplasms of the thymic epithelial cells, regardless of the presence or absence of a lymphoid component." They delegated originality for this concept to BELL [3], who wrote in 1917, "A thymoma may now be defined as a tumor, benign or malignant, probably derived from the thymic epithelium." How one defines the specific phrase "benign or malignant" has remained to this day the premier issue for pathologists and therapists alike.

For therapeutic considerations the thymoma, the commonest tumor of the anterosuperior compartment of the mediastinum, must be presumed to be potentially malignant pending its final surgical/pathologic assessment. Regardless of the presence or absence of symptoms, therefore, the possibility of surgical

EARLE W. WILKINS, JR., M.D., Clinical Professor of Surgery, Emeritus, Harvard Medical School, Massachusetts General Hospital, 32 Fruit Street, Boston, MA 02114, USA

removal must be given priority in any therapeutic sequence. The author prefers to avoid preoperative confirmatory biopsy unless mediastinal contrast-enchanced computed tomography (CT) indicates that total excision of tumor is not likely. There is an apparent propensity for a thymoma to reimplant locally or to metastasize to pleural surfaces if tumor capsule is transgressed surgically or even by needle biopsy.

Overall therapy, particularly in the decision to utilize adjuvant measures postsurgically, depends on assessment of malignancy. MARCHEVSKY and KANEKO [1] state "most encapsulated, benign thymomas have identical histologic and cytologic features to invasive thymomas." ROSAI and LEVINE [2] comment that "the surgeon is usually in a better position to assess the invasive nature of a thymoma from the findings at thoracotomy than the pathologist who examines the specimen after removal." In an earlier study of surgically managed patients with thymoma at the Massachusetts General Hospital, however, the author [4] has concluded that "pathologic staging of thymomas by the method of Masaoka should supplement the gross surgical assessment of encapsulation vs invasion."

There has also been expanding recent interest in the microscopic definition of the malignant potential of thymomas by the classification of Marino and Müller-Hermelink relating thymoma epithelial cells to the medullary and cortical differentiation of the normal thymus [5]. Their current classification of thymic epithelial tumors (the thymoma and thymic carcinoma) includes six subtypes: medullary, mixed, predominantly cortical, cortical, well-differentiated carcinoma, and high-grade carcinomas (epidermoid, undifferentiated, and endocrine thymic carcinomas) [6]. QUINTANILLA-MARTINEZ et al. suggest that this "histologic subclassification is an independent prognostic factor," that is, independent of staging [7, 8].

If either surgical or pathologic staging determines invasion or if the more cortical or frankly carcinomatous differentiation of the thymic epithelial tumor cell is present, the need for adjuvant therapy becomes real. Here again, however, the opportunity for surgical excision of a thymoma must be afforded a primary role unless the tumor is very large and thought by CT to be invasive, in which case radiation therapy, following anterior mediastinotomy biopsy, may be provided first.

2.2 Principles of Surgical Management

The basic principles of surgical management include:

1. Assessment of the extent of the anterosuperior mediastinal tumor by CT utilizing contrast enhancement
2. Avoidance of needle or open biopsy unless the CT extent of tumor indicates complete resection is unlikely
3. Use of a total median sternotomy incision
4. Opening of both pleural sacs for accurate gross estimate of the extent of tumor
5. Total thymectomy including all apparently normal thymus
6. Extended resection of invasive tumors including pericardium, pleura, lung parenchyma, phrenic nerve, or left innominate vein where necessary
7. Excisional stripping of parietal pleural implants

Computed tomographic evaluation of the mediastinum is essential in the planning of surgery for any mediastinal tumor. It constitutes the surgeon's road map to the complex vascular anatomy of the thorax. That is why the injection of contrast material is important in all but small anterior mediastinal tumors or ones in which vascular structures are obviously not compromised. The gross extent of tumor without apparent vascular invasion of other than the left innominate vein is not a contraindication to primary surgical exploration. The presence of enlarged mediastinal lymph nodes on CT examinations suggests that the tumor is a lymphoma and is a contraindication to primary operation without mediastinoscopic assessment of the nodes.

Needle aspiration of an anterior mediastinal tumor not only raises the possibility of implantation of thymoma but often does not provide adequate biopsy material for more than cytologic study. The differentiation of the various lymphomas from thymoma usually is not possible without a block of tissue to provide the pathologist with the opportunity to assess cellular architecture. If there is CT evidence to suggest that complete excision of the tumor is not likely, biopsy can be performed by the anterior mediastinotomy approach of Chamberlain. Conventional mediastinoscopy does not provide access to the anterior mediastinum.

Median sternotomy, the incision of choice, provides optimal access to the thymus gland, wherever within it the thymoma may lie. It is a generally well-tolerated incision. It provides easy approach to any structures needing excision in the extended dissection of an invasive thymoma. It facilitates removal of the entire thymus gland. The cervical approach, on the contrary, provides only limited access. Video-assisted thoracoscopic removal of a thymoma, while technically possible in the small, noninvasive tumor, does not permit an aggressively thorough, clean, and complete dissection of the anterior mediastinum.

Opening the pleural space, particularly on the side of the greater extent of tumor, adds no increased hazard to the operative technique and does facilitate both the proper surgical staging of tumor and the removal of large tumors. It provides irrefutable evidence of the presence or absence of pleural implants.

Total thymectomy is advisable, both because foci of thymoma may lie outside the main tumor within apparently normal thymus and because myasthenia gravis (MG) has been reported to develop after removal of a thymoma [4]. In the latter circumstance, the options of treatment of the MG are simplified by knowing that the thymus gland has been removed.

However malignant, thymomas are usually slow to recur. An aggressive approach to removal of all tumor seems justified in those cases where extended resections permit removal of all gross tumor. Care must be taken in the decision to remove a phrenic nerve. In the nonmyasthenic patient, this is usually well tolerated; in the myasthenic, it may make respirator weaning difficult. The author does not see advantage in debulking tumor per se. Stripping pleural implants of thymoma, on the other hand, is an easy addendum to surgery which can be accomplished without appreciable risk with the pleural sac already opened and the parietal pleura exposed.

Again, special note is made concerning very large tumors. If biopsy by anterior mediastinotomy is elected as the initial procedure, preoperative radiation therapy to a dose of 30–45 Gy represents the treatment of choice, both to decrease the size of the tumor for ease of resection and to minimize mediastinal or transpleural seeding of tumor. This may be followed in 3–4 weeks by median sternotomy and tumor removal.

2.3 Staging

Neither surgical nor pathologic staging of thymoma was available before Bergh's report in 1978 [9]. The Masaoka modification [10] has now become the standard clinical staging system.

- Stage I. Macroscopically completely encapsulated with no microscopic extracapsular invasion
- Stage II. Microscopic invasion through the capsule or macroscopic invasion of the mediastinal fatty tissue or mediastinal pleura
- Stage III. Macroscopic invasion into adjacent structure (i.e., pericardium, great vessels, or lung)
- Stage IVA. Pleural or pericardial dissemination
- Stage IVB. Lymphatic or hematogenous metastasis

In the series following, the author has added the refinement of classifying the finding of foci of tumor within otherwise normal thymus as stage II and macroscopic invasion of a phrenic nerve as stage III. No attempt has been made to break down stages II and III into A and B depending on microscopic (A) or gross (B) invasion. Such subclassification seems arbitrary.

2.4 The MGH Experience

The 20-year period from 1972 to 1992 at the Massachusetts General Hospital (MGH) has been chosen for evaluation. All patients studied were on the General Thoracic Surgical Service and were cared for by cardiothoracic residents in training under the supervision of attending general thoracic surgeons. This period of time coincides with the era when MG was neither a determinant in long-term survival of patients with thymoma nor a major factor in postoperative morbidity.

A diagnosis of thymoma was made in 103 patients in this period. This represents 55% of the overall MGH experience of 186 patients from 1939 to 1992.

2.4.1 Demographics

There were 52 females and 51 males. Their ages ranged from a 13-year-old girl to an 84-year-old male. The distribution comprised all intervening decades and is detailed in Table 2.1, where the peak incidence in males is seen to be between ages 40 and 59 (22 cases), but in females between 60 and 79 (30 cases).

Table 2.1. Incidence of thymoma in 103 patients listed by decade of age and gender

Age	Male	Female	Total
10–19	1	2	3
20–29	2	2	4
30–39	8	4	12
40–49	12	2	14
50–59	10	11	21
60–69	7	18	25
70–79	8	12	20
80–89	3	1	4
	51	52	103

Myasthenia gravis was present in 21 males and 14 females. In addition, symptoms of MG were first detected post-thymomectomy in two males. The total of 37 MG patients represents 36% of all 103 thymoma patients, a decrease from the 59% in the first 63 patients reported from the MGH [11]. Except for the 13-year-old female and an 18-year-old male, all thymomas in MG patients occurred over 30 years of age.

2.4.2 Presenting Symptoms

In the 35 patients presenting with MG (27 systemic, eight ocular), the diagnosis of thymoma was suggested by chest roentgenography. Among the 68 other patients, the tumor was detected on a routine chest radiograph in 23 and by a film taken for investigation of a nonthoracic problem in 12 others. In the remaining 33 patients the chief complaint was chest pain in 16, persisting cough in eight, dyspnea in four, intercurrent respiratory infection in three, and pure red blood cell aplasia and hypogammaglobulinemia in one each. These were the only instances, other than MG, representing autoimmune disease. In summary, approximately one-third of these thymoma patients had MG, one-third had other symptoms related to the tumor, and one-third had tumors which were asymptomatic.

2.4.3 Preoperative Diagnosis

Following a long-held MGH dictum shunning preoperative tissue confirmation for fear of local implantation of thymoma, 90 patients were operated upon de novo, that is without a positive diagnosis or a biopsy attempt. In nine patients definitive tissue diagnosis was obtained by a limited anterior mediastinotomy (the Chamberlain technique). Two of these cases were deemed unresectable and had no further surgery. In three patients mediastinoscopy was performed with establishment of definitive pathologic diagnosis in two. Subsequent resection was carried out in all three. Needle aspiration biopsy, attempted in five patients, yielded a tissue diagnosis in none. One patient had a positive diagnosis provided by the Vim-Silverman needle method. This was her only surgical procedure because of a precarious general medical status.

2.4.4 Operations

An attempt at thymectomy was carried out in 100 patients, by a median sternotomy in 96 and by lateral thoracotomy in four patients. Gross tumor removal was possible in 97, subtotal removal in two, and biopsy only in one. In the remaining three patients a Chamberlain anterior mediastinotomy biopsy was the only surgery in two and the Vim-Silverman needle biopsy, the only surgery in one.

Extended resection for invasive thymoma was necessary in 23 patients. The tissue removed beyond thymus gland and mediastinal fat included pericardium in 19 patients, lung in 14 (wedge excision in 12, lobectomy in two), a single phrenic nerve in ten, the innominate vein in five, pleural implants in two, and chest wall in one.

2.4.5 Staging

Final Masaoka staging is presented in Table 2.2, which compares the surgeon's gross operating staging with the pathologist's microscopic evaluation. The pathologist's assessment of microscopic invasion resulted in upgrading the surgeon's stage from I to II in 13 cases and from II to III in four cases. This is further confirmation of the primary conclusion in the WILKINS et al. report in 1991 that pathologic microscopic evaluation should supplement surgical gross appraisal in the final determination of stage [4].

2.4.6 Pathology

There has been a spate of recent papers in the general thoracic and pathology literature on the Marino and Müller-Hermelink classification of thymoma and

Table 2.2. A comparison of gross and microscopic staging (numbers refer to number of patients)

Stage	Surgical gross	Pathologic microscopic
I	55	42
II	21	30
III	23	27
IVA	3	3
IVB	1	1
	103	103

Table 2.3. Correlation of histologic subtyping[a] and clinicopathologic staging

Histologic subtype	Stage				
	I	II	III	IVA	IVB
Medullary (11)	8	3			
Mixed (29)	18	11			
Predominantly cortical (17)	8	7	2		
Cortical (12)	5	4	3		
Well-differentiated carcinoma (25)		5	16	3	1
High-grade carcinoma (2)			2		
	39	30	23	3	1

[a] Subtyping could not be applied in two cases. One specimen (surgically graded stage I) was necrotic following preoperative radiation; a second (surgically graded stage III) was infracted

thymic carcinoma which relates thymoma epithelial cells to the cortical and medullary differentiation of the thymus gland [5,6]. With the aid of Professor Müller-Hermelink, who visited the MGH in 1991, instructing the pathology staff in the use of his classification and reviewing all histologic material, 98 of the 103 cases have been categorized into this newer histologic subclassification. Slides and paraffin blocks were not available in five cases earlier in this 20-year review. A comparison of histologic subtyping with clinicopathologic staging is presented in Table 2.3. All patients with medullary (Fig. 2.1) or mixed thymomas were stage I (65%) or II (35%). Most patients with well-differentiated (Fig. 2.2) or high-grade carcinoma were stage III and IV (80% and 100% respectively). Those with predominantly cortical (Fig. 2.3) and cortical thymomas showed intermediate invasion; 45% were stage I, 38% stage II, and 17% stage III.

2.4.7 Results

There was one perioperative death in this series of 103 patients with thymoma, an 84-year-old male

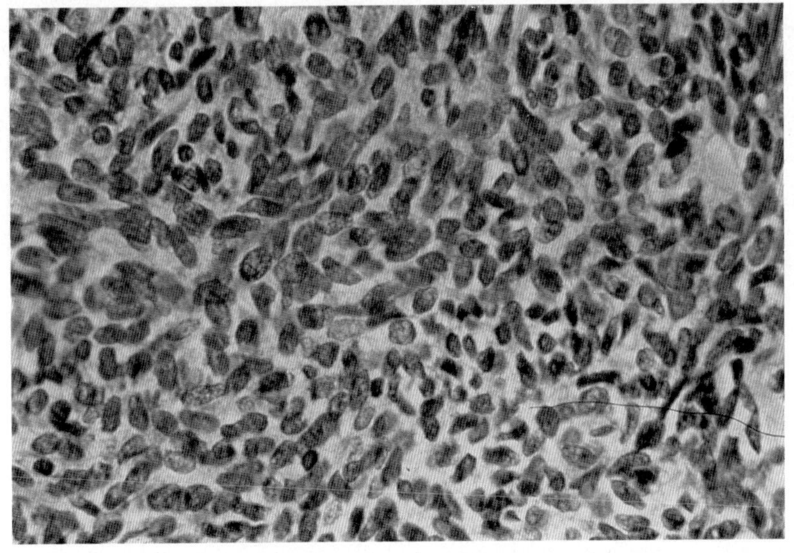

Fig. 2.1. Photomicrograph of a medullary thymoma with spindled cells. Some medullary thymomas have oval or round cells forming rosettes or gland-like spaces. Lymphocytes are uncommon

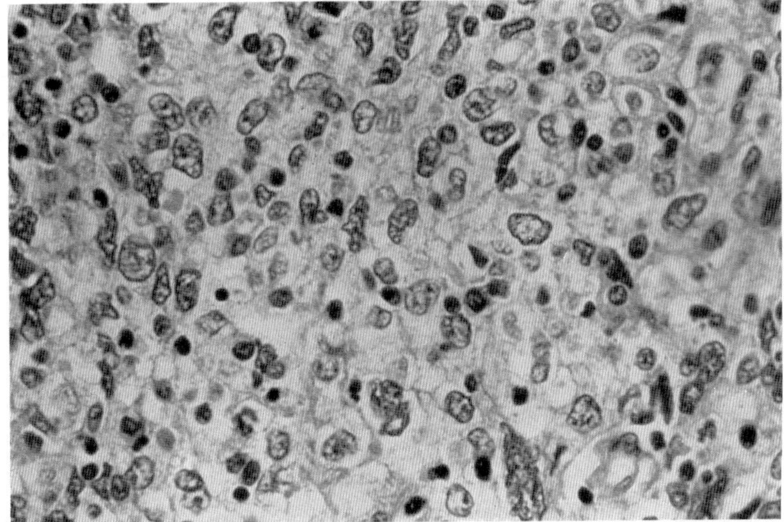

Fig. 2.2. Photomicrograph of a well-differentiated carcinoma with features of scarce lymphocytes, cytologic atypia and mitotic activity

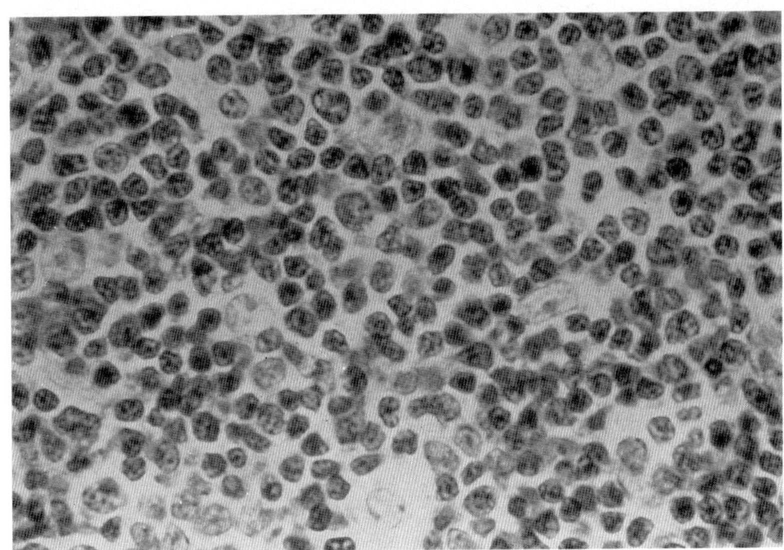

Fig. 2.3. Photomicrograph of a predominantly cortical thymoma resembling very closely the cytology and architecture of normal thymus. QUINTANILLA-MARTINEZ et al. [7] propose the term "organoid" thymoma

who died on his 45th postoperative day from multiorgan failure stemming from respiratory insufficiency. His pathology was, tragically, only stage I disease. One patient has been lost to follow-up.

Of the remaining 101 patients, 21 have died, 12 of unrelated causes, six from recurrent or persisting thymoma, two from myasthenic crisis with respiratory failure, and one by suicide. The timing of the late mortality in these 21 cases is recorded in Table 2.4. A most important finding is that, of the 80 patients known to be alive, four have developed recurrence of thymoma. All of these had, in the opinion of the operating surgeon, total gross removal of tumor:

Case 1. A male with MG, stage II well-differentiated carcinoma, developed recurrence of tumor at 6 years, requiring a left pleuropneumonectomy followed by radiation, and is alive free of disease at 10 years.

Case 2. A female with MG, stage II well-differentiated carcinoma, developed recurrence of tumor at 5 years, underwent a re-resection, and is alive with further recurrence at 8 years.

Case 3. A woman with stage III well-differentiated carcinoma developed recurrence of tumor in her eighth year, had a left pneumonectomy, and is alive, apparently without disease, at 10 years.

Case 4. A woman with MG originally considered stage I but reevaluated as stage II when she was given the histologic predominantly cortical subtyping developed recurrence of tumor at 13 years, underwent re-resection, and is free of disease 1 year later.

None of those four patients underwent postoperative radiation therapy, because of the surgeon's operative gross assessment that all tumor had been removed.

Actuarial survival, as clarified by GRUNKEMEIER and STARR [12], was calculated for 85 patients operated upon prior to 1990. The overall survival was 64% at 10 years; the figure for stage I disease was 78%, for stage II, 75%, and for stage III, only 21%. This is presented graphically in Fig. 2.4 with the difference between the overlapping curves for stages I–II and the curve for stage III significant to a *P* factor of 0.0001 [4].

2.4.8 Adjuvant Therapy

Radiation therapy was not utilized per specific protocol. It was used for 33 patients in doses ranging from 30 to 60 Gy: in 13 of 21 stage II patients, in 17 of 23 stage III patients, and in all three stage IVA patients. It was employed preoperatively in one

Table 2.4. Late mortality

Stage	Within postoperative interval:		
	1 year	5 years	10 years
I	1	2	2
II		1	2
III	2 (2)	4 (3)	3 (1)
IVA			2 (2)
IVB	1 (1)		

[a] The numbers in parentheses indicate deaths from thymoma (6), myasthenia gravis (2) and suicide (1). An additional stage I patient died at 12 years of an unrelated cause

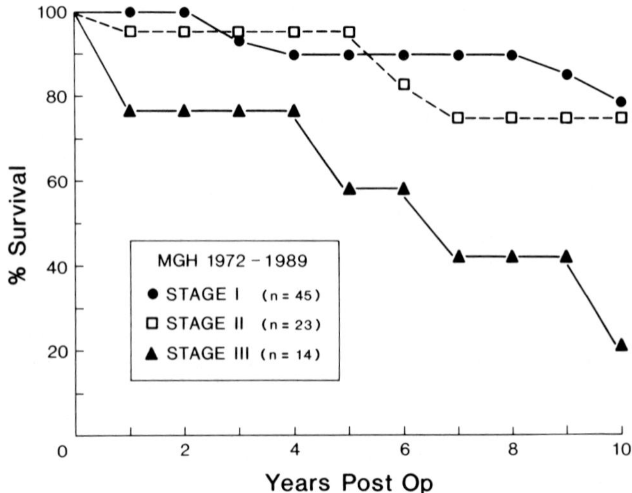

Fig. 2.4. Actuarial survival vs pathologic staging of thymoma (stages I and II vs III). (From [4])

stage II and one stage III patient, and both preoperatively and postoperatively in another stage III patient. Because of variation of dosage and lack of standard application of therapy in stage II patients, no attempt is made to draw conclusions on the effectiveness of radiation therapy in this series.

Chemotherapy was given to three patients, again not according to standard protocol. All were patients with well-differentiated thymic carcinoma, one each in stages III, IVA, and IVB. It proved ineffective in all.

2.5 Discussion

There seems to be room for controversy in only two areas involving thymomas. The first is in the definition. Although PESCARMOMA and associates [13] excluded "tumors that displayed clear-cut malignant histological features, i.e., thymic carcinoma," it would seem preferable to include all tumors of the thymic epithelial cell and avoid any confusion by using Müller-Hermelink's all-inclusive term "thymoma and thymic carcinoma." All are thymic tumors and typically unknown in relative malignancy until removed. In the present review the newer histologic subclassification of thymomas has been helpful as an independent prognostic factor. It has been suggested by WICK [14] and KORNSTEIN [15], however, that the classification, in its complexity, will not replace staging as the major prognostic factor for patients with thymoma.

The second area for controversy lies in the indications for utilization of adjuvant radiation therapy. Here a further look at results in the MGH series may be helpful. (The staging numbers are those determined by microscopy.)

Stage I: The 42 stage I patients were all managed with thymectomy alone according to the basic surgical principles earlier expressed. No stage I thymoma patient, whichever the cell type, has experienced tumor relapse or died of thymoma.

Stage II: Three of the 30 stage II patients developed recurrence of thymoma. The tumor cell type was predominantly cortical in one and well-differentiated carcinoma in two. No medullary or mixed stage II thymoma has recurred.

Stage III: The four stage III thymoma patients dying with relapse of their tumor all had well-differentiated carcinoma. The remaining one of the patients alive with recurrence also had well-differentiated carcinoma. Of the 27 stage III patients, only

those with well-differentiated or high-grade carcinoma have relapsed. There were no medullary or mixed tumors in patients with stage III disease (see Table 2.3).

Utilizing these observations, adjuvant radiation therapy would appear unnecessary in any stage I patient and in those stage II patients with medullary or mixed thymomas. Radiation would seem strongly advisable in all other stage II patients and should be an integral part of therapy for all stage III and IVA patients.

An area meriting discussion is when to employ preoperative radiation. This is more a matter of judgment than controversy. The Toronto group report in 1984 speculated that the use of preoperative radiation in large, possibly invasive thymomas would reduce tumor bulk, permitting easier dissection, and "prevent transpleural metastatic seeding at the time of operation" [16]. Although preoperative radiation was utilized in only two patients in the MGH series reported, this approach has considerable appeal. It does mandate the need for preradiation biopsy.

A final area for discussion is the admittedly arbitrary avoidance of routine preoperative biopsy of a thymoma. The obvious problem is how one knows that an anterior mediastinal tumor is indeed a thymoma. If CT study fails to demonstrate mediastinal adenopathy, characteristic of lymphomas, where primary surgery is not the treatment of choice, a direct surgical attack is desirable, both for thymoma and for other nonlymphomatous tumors of the area.

The discussion would not be complete without comment on thymoma patients with MG. Such patients are prepared for surgery, preferably with plasmapheresis if the MG is severe. The possibly adverse effects of sacrifice of a phrenic nerve should be very carefully considered before proceeding therewith. Postoperative care is optimally carried out in a respiratory care unit avoiding anticholinesterase therapy for 48–72 h. Long-term results of thymoma therapy seem not to be adversely affected by the presence of MG. It is probably no more than coincidence that three of the four living patients with thymoma recurrence have MG. Relief of myasthenic symptoms must not be expected in patients undergoing total thymectomy with removal of the thymoma. MAGGI et al. [17], in a report of 241 cases of thymoma, found that the prognosis in patients with MG and thymoma was actually more favorable than in patients without MG, possibly the result of earlier detection. The comparison of histologic subtyping and staging in MG patients is illustrated in Table 2.5.

Table 2.5. Histologic subtyping and clinicopathologic staging in 34 MG patients

Histologic subtype	Stage			
	I	II	III	IVA
Medullary (2)	2			
Mixed (6)	5	1		
Predominantly cortical (8)	5	3		
Cortical (9)	4	5		
Well-differentiated carcinoma (9)		3	5	1

2.6 Summary

1. Surgical dissection and removal is the primary therapeutic management for thymoma.
2. Contrast-enhanced CT is the principal investigative method in the evaluation of thymoma.
3. Preoperative biopsy confirmation of thymoma is unnecessary, perhaps even contraindicated, in most patients with thymoma.
4. If the tumor is very large or possibly unresectable by CT, anterior mediastinotomy biopsy and preoperative radiation constitute a reasonable alternative to direct primary surgery.
5. Pathologic staging by the criteria of Masaoka must supplement gross surgical assessment of encapsulation of tumor vs invasion.
6. The Marino, Müller-Hermelink and Kirchner histologic subclassification should prove to be a reliable independent prognostic factor.
7. No stage I, or medullary or mixed thymoma, has recurred in the MGH series. Further therapy is unnecessary for these patients.
8. All patients in stage III or with well-differentiated carcinoma by histologic classification are candidates for postresection radiation therapy.
9. Stage II patients, or those with predominantly cortical or cortical tumors, constitute an intermediate group in which a few tumors have recurred. Postoperative radiation should be carefully considered and probably advised.
10. Thymoma patients are at risk for late tumor recurrence and should be carefully followed at yearly intervals at least until 10 years. The 10-year actuarial survival is the standard for measuring outcome.

References

1. Marchevsky AM, Kaneko M (1984) Surgical pathology of the mediastinum. Raven Press, New York, pp 58–116
2. Rosai J, Levine GD (1976) Tumors of the thymus. Atlas of tumor pathology, fascicle 13, second series, Armed Forces Institute of Pathology, Washington DC, pp 34–161
3. Bell ET (1917) Tumors of the thymus in myasthenia gravis. J Nerv Ment Dis 45: 130–143
4. Wilkins EW Jr, Grillo HC, Scannell JG, Moncure AC, Mathisen DJ (1991) Role of staging in prognosis and management of thymoma. Ann Thorac Surg 51: 888–892
5. Marino M, Müller-Hermelink HK (1985) Thymoma and thymic carcinoma. Relation of thymoma epithelial cells to the cortical and medullary differentiation of thymus. Virchows Arch [A] 407: 119–149
6. Kirchner T, Müller-Hermelink HK (1989) New approaches to the diagnosis of thymic epithelial tumors. Prog Surg Pathol 10: 167–189
7. Quintanilla-Martinez L, Müller-Hermelink HK, Wilkins EW Jr, Ferry JA, Harris NL (1993) Thymoma: histogenetic subclassification correlates with clinical and immunohistochemical features. A study of 122 cases. Hum Pathol 24: 958–969
8. Quintanilla-Martinez L, Wilkins EW Jr, Efird JT, Hug E, Choi NC, Harris NL (1994) Thymoma: histologic subclassification is an independent prognostic factor. Cancer 74: 606–617
9. Bergh NP, Gatzinsky P, Larsson S, Lundin P, Rindell B (1978) Tumors of the thymus and thymic region. I. Clinicopathologic studies on thymomas. Ann Thorac Surg 25: 91–98
10. Masaoka A, Monden Y, Nakahara K, Tanioka T (1981) Follow-up study of thymoma with special reference to their clinical stages. Cancer 48: 2485–2492
11. Wilkins EW Jr, Edmunds LH Jr, Castleman B (1966) Cases of thymoma at the Massachusetts General Hospital. J Thorac Cardiovasc Surg 52: 322–330
12. Grunkemeier GI, Starr A (1977) Actuarial analysis of surgical results: rationale and method. Ann Thorac Surg 24: 404–408
13. Pescarmona E, Rendina EA, Venuta F, et al. (1990) Analysis of prognostic factors and clinicopathological staging of thymoma. Ann Thorac Surg 50: 534–538
14. Wick MR (1990) Assessing the prognosis of thymomas. Ann Thorac Surg 50: 521–522
15. Kornstein MJ (1992) Controversies regarding the pathology of thymomas. Pathol Ann: 1–15
16. Shamji F, Pearson FG, Todd TRJ, Ginsberg RJ, Ilves R, Cooper JD (1984) Results of surgical treatment for thymoma. J Thorac Cardiovasc Surg 87: 43–47
17. Maggi G, Casadio C, Cavallo A, Cianci R, Molinatti M, Ruffini E (1991) Thymoma: results of 241 operated cases. Ann Thorac Surg 51: 152–156

3 Thymoma: Radiation and Chemotherapy

WUI-JIN KOH, PATRICK J. LOEHRER, SR., and CHARLES R. THOMAS, JR.

CONTENTS

3.1 Introduction

The initial treatment of choice for all thymomas, with the exception of rare cases presenting with grossly unresectable local disease or diffuse metastases, is complete tumor resection. Surgical considerations are discussed elsewhere in this volume [1]. While various investigators have suggested that histological morphology [2–5] and flow cytometric assessment [6] may have prognostic implications, the primary determinants of clinical outcome are surgicopathologic staging and the related extent of surgical resection [7–10], which then form the basis for selection of adjuvant radiation and/or chemotherapy.

Historically, a thymoma has been considered "benign" or "malignant" on the basis of surgical assessment of tumor encapsulation or invasiveness. Clinical staging for thymoma was first introduced by BERGH et al. [11] in 1978, and was subsequently modified by MASAOKA et al. [12] in 1981 to

WUI-JIN KOH, M.D., Associate Professor, Department of Radiation Oncology, University of Washington, RC-08, Seattle, WA 98195 USA
PATRICK J. LOEHRER, SR., M.D., Professor of Medicine, Section of Hematology and Oncology, Indiana University School of Medicine, Indianapolis, IN 46202-2879, USA
CHARLES R. THOMAS, JR., M.D., Fellow, Department of Radiation Oncology, University of Washington Medical Center, RC-08, 1959 NE Pacific Street, Seattle, WA 98195, USA

include greater emphasis on histologic evaluation (Table 3.1). Other investigators have adapted the Bergh and/or Masaoka criteria in single-institution reports [3, 13, 14]. The Masaoka classification, with various minor modifications, is currently the most widely used staging system. In addition to its inclusion of a fourth stage, it should be noted that the Masaoka scheme is more stringent than the Bergh system for determination of stage I disease. Patients with Bergh stage I tumors who have microscopic invasion into, but not through, the capsule would be considered Masaoka stage II. Recently, a TNM system, based almost entirely on the Masaoka scheme, has been proposed [15].

3.2 Radiation Therapy

It is difficult to compare the results of different studies and define stage-related adjuvant treatment algorithms. Some of the reasons include the relative rarity of thymomas, the often indolent natural history of these tumors, the disparate staging systems used, and the application of these staging criteria retrospectively to clinical experiences accrued over extended time intervals. This is especially true for patients with invasive thymomas, which encompass stage II–IV disease according to the Masaoka staging system.

The percentage of complete tumor resectability has varied among different series, depending on patient selection and surgical experience. Patients who are considered to have undergone subtotal resection have had variable amounts of residual disease, ranging from microscopic residual to nearly the entire presenting gross tumor volume. Postoperative radiotherapy has not been administered in a systematic manner, and, when prescribed, has included a broad range of doses and varying treatment techniques. No prospective trials of adjuvant or primary radiotherapy have been carried out. Local control and distant failure have often been poorly documented, and not specifically correlated

Table 3.1. Clinicopathologic staging systems for thymoma

BERGH et al. [11]

Stage I:	Intact capsule or growth within the capsule
Stage II:	Pericapsular growth into the mediastinal fat tissue
Stage III:	Invasive growth into the surrounding organs, intrathoracic metastases, or both

MASAOKA et al. [12]

Stage I:	Macroscopically completely encapsulated and microscopically no capsular invasion
Stage II:	1. Macroscopic invasion into surrounding fatty tissue or mediastinal pleura, *or* 2. Microscopic invasion into capsule
Stage III:	Macroscopic invasion into neighboring organ, i.e., pericardium, great vessels, or lung
Stage IVa:	Pleural or pericardial dissemination
Stage IVb:	Lymphogenous or hematogenous metastasis

with tumor stage, extent of surgery, and postoperative irradiation. Furthermore, several studies have related effectiveness of thymoma treatment to control of myasthenic symptoms rather than actual tumor outcome [16].

Finally, recent substantial advances in surgery, anesthesiology, diagnostic radiology, and radiation oncology provide for better staging, resection, and radiotherapy, thereby limiting the comparability of information from either clinical series. Nevertheless, through a survey of the existing literature, some guidelines may be provided on the role of radiotherapy in the management of thymomas.

3.2.1 Encapsulated Thymomas

By definition, all encapsulated thymomas are completely resectable, with the possible exception of the extremely rare instance when a bulky tumor is ruptured at the time of surgery [17]. This group of patients include those with stage I tumors in both the Bergh and Masaoka classifications, as well as some with Masaoka stage II disease who have *no evidence of tumor beyond the capsule*. The importance of careful pathologic review in addition to surgical assessment of capsular invasion has been emphasized, with reported pathologic upstaging occurring in more than 10% of patients [10]. While a few investigators have advocated routine postoperative radiation for all patients with thymomas regardless of stage [7], it is well recognized that the risk of failure following complete resection of encapsulated disease is very low, and most would agree that adjuvant therapy is not indicated for such

patients, in whom disease-specific survival rates approach 100%. Table 3.2 shows the cumulative experience with complete surgical resection *alone* in patients with encapsulated thymomas, with an overall intrathoracic failure rate of 3%. However, it has been emphasized that since thymomas tend to be slow-growing tumors, follow-up should be continued for a minimum of 10 years [10]. For the rare failures, aggressive radiotherapy can be incorporated into multimodal approaches for attempted salvage [25].

3.2.2 Completely Resected Invasive Disease (Stages II and III)

This heterogeneous category of patients includes those with Masaoka stages II, III, and, rarely, IVa disease. The rate of complete resectability varies by stage (essentially 100% for stage II, 50%–60% for stage III, and very infrequently for stage IVa tumors) [7, 9, 14, 22–24, 26].

Many authors recommend adjuvant radiotherapy following total surgical resection of invasive thymomas. CURRAN and colleagues [14] strongly suggest the need for postoperative thoracic irradiation in such patients. In 21 patients with completely resected thymomas (18 stage II and 3 stage III) who did not undergo postoperative irradiation, eight mediastinal failures were noted, for a crude local failure rate of 38%, a 5-year actuarial mediastinal relapse rate of 53%, and a 5-year relapse-free survival rate of 47%. By comparison, there were no failures among five patients (one stage II and four stage III) who received adjuvant radiotherapy, and these patients had a 5-year relapse-free survival rate of 100%. CURRAN et al. also pooled their data with those from seven other studies [18, 19, 21, 27–30] in which patients underwent complete resection of invasive stage II and III thymomas. Overall, the combined experience revealed a crude 28% (20/72) intrathoracic failure rate in patients who did not receive postoperative radiotherapy, versus a 5% (2/43) failure rate in irradiated cases [14].

The usefulness of adjuvant radiotherapy following complete resection of stage III thymomas is further supported by URGESI and co-workers, who noted that in 33 such patients, there were no in-field recurrences, although there were three out-of-field intrathoracic relapses. However, there was no surgery-only group for comparison [26]. ARAKAWA and co-workers reported 15 patients with invasive thymomas (stages III and IV) who received postop-

Table 3.2. Completely resected stage I thymoma, without adjuvant treatment

Series	No. of patients	No. failed	Follow-up interval	Comments	Staging system
BATATA et al. 1974 [18]	18	0	Range: 5–17 yrs		NA
NORDSTROM et al. 1979 [19]	25	1	Up to 10 yrs	Recurrence at 4 years, salvaged with radiation	B
APPELQVIST et al. 1982 [20]	17	0	Up to 10 yrs		NA
VERLEY and HOLLMANN 1985 [3]	133	7	Median $\sim$ 10 yrs	All recurrences by 7.7 years	M
MAGGI et al. 1986 [21]	106	4	Median 5 yrs	Recurrences from 3 to 8 years	NA
CURRAN et al. 1988 [14]	41	0	Median 4.1 yrs	Included 7 patients with adhesions between the thymoma and adjacent structures, but no pathologic tumor invasion through the capsule	B
NAKAHARA et al. 1988 [7]	14	1	Up to 15 yrs	Recurrence at 4 years	M
WILKINS et al. 1991 [10]	45	0	Up to 10 yrs		M
HANIUDA et al. 1992 [22]	17	0	Up to 15 yrs		M
POLLACK et al. 1992 [23]	5	1	Median 46 months	Recurrence at 30 months	M
ETIENNE et al. 1993 [24]	13	0	Mean 11.2 yrs		M
Total	434	14			

B, Bergh staging system; M, Masaoka staging system; NA, not available – staging system not specified, with thymoma considered stage I on basis of reported absence of extracapsular invasion

erative radiotherapy following total surgical extirpation. Only two tumor recurrences were noted, and all patients remained alive at last follow-up [16]. NAKAHARA et al. noted a 95% 15-year survival rate in 35 patients with stage III thymomas who were completely resected and given routine postoperative radiation [7]. These results support the standard use, at present, of postoperative radiotherapy following complete surgical resection of stage III disease. Local adjuvant treatment (i.e., radiotherapy) for the very rare patient with completely resected stage IVa thymoma may perhaps be inferred from results in stage III tumors.

While there is general consensus regarding the use of adjuvant radiotherapy in fully resected stage III disease, its role in invasive stage II thymoma (tumor extending through the capsule into mediastinal fat) is more widely debated. In the experience of CURRAN et al., six of 18 completely resected stage II tumors in patients who did not receive radiotherapy eventually recurred in the mediastinum as the first site of relapse [14]. MONDEN et al. reported a 29% (2/7) recurrence rate for patients with resected stage II thymomas who did not undergo adjuvant irradiation, as compared to 8% (2/25) in those who received postoperative radiotherapy [29]. Other investigators have noted a low rate of recurrence in completely resected stage II disease and questioned the need for routine radiotherapy [9, 26].

WILKINS reported three recurrences in 30 patients with stage II thymomas following complete tumor removal. He emphasized the importance of adding histologic criteria to surgicopathologic staging in assessing prognosis for these patients, since recurrences occurred in patients with more aggressive histologic profiles (one with predominantly cortical thymoma and two with well-differentiated carcinomas). While his observations may support limiting the use of adjunctive radiotherapy to patients with more "histologically aggressive" stage II tumors, it should be noted that approximately one-third of the stage II patients received postoperative radiotherapy, making definitive conclusions difficult [1]. PESCARMONA et al. have presented a rather complex scheme of combined clinicopathologic staging, which supports the recommendations of Wilkins in using postoperative radiotherapy only for selected patients with stage II thymomas [4]. An intriguing suggestion involving pathologic evaluation of a "pleural factor" has been made by HANIUDA and colleagues as a potentially useful guide to the selection of postoperative radiation in patients with completely resected stage II thymomas, i.e., those with fibrous adhesions or microscopic invasion to the mediastinal pleura are at increased risk for recurrence and may benefit from adjuvant therapy [22].

Despite the varying opinions expressed by different investigators, it is our recommendation that, pending further clinical validation of proposed prognostic factors, postoperative radiotherapy be considered in all patients with completely resected stage II thymomas when tumor extension beyond the capsule is documented pathologically.

3.2.3 Incompletely Resected Local-Regionally Extensive Tumors

This category consists primarily of patients with Masaoka stage III and IVa thymomas. Surgical approaches used in this population range from biopsy alone to near-complete tumor removal, making comparisons between different series difficult [14, 17, 21, 23].

Thymomas are moderately radiosensitive, and radical postoperative radiotherapy, typically described as doses ≥ 40 Gy, can control residual disease and provide long-term disease-free survival in patients with incompletely resected tumors. Table 3.3 provides a summary of clinical experiences where approximate 5-year data are available: the overall crude local control and survival rates are 65% (166/255) and 45% (49/109), respectively. More recent series have reported data in actuarial terms, but these remain in close agreement, with 5-year survival rates of about 40%–50% [3, 7, 9, 23, 26, 32].

The extent of residual disease preradiation has a significant impact on tumor control and survival. JACKSON and BALL reported 28 patients with incompletely resected thymomas who received postoperative radiotherapy. Among 14 patients for whom gross tumor removal was possible, leaving only microscopic residual, local control was achieved in 13 (93%), and the 10-year overall actuarial survival rate was 62%. In comparison, 14 other patients had gross residual tumor, with a local control rate of 4/14 (29%) and a 10-year survival rate of 29% [17]. POLLACK and colleagues reported an actuarial 5-year disease-free survival rate of 60% following radiotherapy in subtotally resected thymomas (defined as removal of $\geq 50\%$ but $< 100\%$ of the tumor), as compared to 20% for patients who had tumor biopsies only ($< 50\%$ of disease surgically removed) [23].

Other authors have also described better clinical outcomes with more aggressive tumor debulking in patients with incompletely resectable thymomas [7, 9, 12, 26]. Given the limited experience of any single institution and the lack of prospective multicenter data, there is an expected selection bias in the reports of better outcome with radical tumor debulking, in that patients with stage III or less bulky thymomas are more likely to have greater resectability than patients with stage IVa or more extensive tumors. However, it would seem appropriate to recommend maximal operative debulking, commensurate with safe surgical principles, even in patients with incompletely resectable disease, who are then candidates for radical postoperative radiotherapy.

Despite aggressive surgery and radiotherapy, patients with regionally advanced stage III and IV thymomas remain at substantial risk of relapse, both locally and distantly. Up to one-third of patients with locally advanced tumors will develop distant extrathoracic failures [14, 32, 33, 39]. The incorporation of chemotherapy into the multimodal management of such patients deserves further study (see below).

3.2.4 Radiotherapy Doses and Techniques

A wide variety of techniques, doses, and fractionation schemes have been utilized over the years. Typically, a dose of 40–50 Gy, in conventional frac-

Table 3.3. Incompletely resected invasive thymoma treated with radical radiotherapy

Series	No. of evaluable patients	No. locally controlled	No. of survivors[a]
PENN and HOPE-STONE 1972 [30]	2	NA	2
MARKS et al. 1978 [28]	6	6	4
ARIARATNAM et al. 1979 [31]	8	5	5
MASAOKA et al. 1981 [12]	19	7	9
ARRIAGADA et al. 1984 [32]	50	34	NA
COHEN et al. 1984 [33]	10	NA	3
KERSH et al. 1985 [34]	10	6	3
VERLEY and HOLLMANN 1985 [3]	29	22	NA
CURRAN et al. 1988 [14]	20	16	NA
KRUEGER et al. 1988 [35]	11	7	3
ARAKAWA et al. 1990 [16]	15	10	8
URGESI et al. 1990 [26]	44	26	NA
JACKSON and BALL 1991 [17]	28	17	12
POLLACK et al. 1992 [23]	15	10	NA
Total	267	166/255	49/109

NA, crude data not available
[a] Five-year survival (approximate)

tionation of about 2 Gy/day, is recommended for adjuvant treatment of completely resected invasive thymomas. Higher doses of up to 60 Gy or even higher have been used for patients with gross residual disease. External beam radiation port arrangements used include a single anterior field, weighted opposed anterior-posterior ports, wedged-pair techniques, and other multiple-field arrangements. Given present technical capabilities, at least two fields, treated daily, are recommended to provide dose homogeneity and allow sparing of adjacent normal critical structures.

Computed tomography is currently indispensable for adequate radiation treatment planning. Clips placed at the time of surgery, either denoting the extent of resection in completely removed thymomas or outlining regions of unresectable disease, are very useful in guiding postoperative radiotherapy. The volume covered should include the entire mediastinum and the adjacent lung and pericardium [36]. For more extensive tumors, various authors have recommended coverage of the supraclavicular nodes [23, 27, 32] and even the entire ipsilaterally involved hemithorax [31, 37]. The incorporation of three-dimensional treatment planning promises further enhancement of radiotherapeutic management through improved tumor dose localization [38].

3.3 Chemotherapy

The role of chemotherapy in the management of thymoma is even less well defined than that of radiation. A large number of drug regimens, employing both single-agent chemotherapy and multiagent combinations, have been reported, but results have mostly been anecdotal in nature. An in-depth review of chemotherapy for thymoma has recently been published [39].

From the standpoint of assessing single-agent activity, only two drugs have been prospectively evaluated in a phase I/II manner, with the remaining information derived from case reports and retrospective reviews. When earlier small series suggested the efficacy of cisplatin in the treatment of advanced thymoma, the Eastern Cooperative Oncology Group (ECOG) conducted a phase II trial using cisplatin (50 mg/m^2 every 3 weeks for a maximum of eight cycles) in patients with metastatic or recurrent thymomas. Twenty patients were fully evaluable. While reasonably well tolerated, there were no complete responses and only two (10%) partial responses. The ECOG concluded that this regimen

of single-agent cisplatin was relatively ineffective in producing tumor regression in this patient population [40].

Recently, a multicenter trial in England has reported efficacy with the use of single-agent ifosfamide (7.5 mg/m^2 every 3 weeks for up to six cycles) in the management of advanced thymomas. Of 13 evaluable patients, seven (54%) achieved a complete response, including two in whom pathologic confirmation was obtained through "second-look" thoracotomy and multiple biopsies following chemotherapy. The complete responses have been durable, ranging from 6 to 66 months, with a median duration of 38 months. One other patient (8%) achieved a partial response, and the remaining five (38%) had stable disease while on chemotherapy. The authors concluded that the reported activity of ifosfamide in malignant thymoma justified its use as a single agent in the first-line therapy for advanced disease [41].

Corticosteroids have also been reported in retrospective series to have activity against thymoma. However, the effectiveness of this class of pharmacologic agents is obscured by the fact that thymoma responses to corticosteroids are typically noted in patients with lymphocyte-predominant histologies, whereas it has been shown that it is the epithelial component of thymoma that represents the malignant cell population [39].

In the pre-cisplatin era, the most commonly used drugs in multi-agent regimens included cyclophosphamide, doxorubicin, and vincristine [39, 42, 43]. More recently, cisplatin has often been incorporated into combination chemotherapy for advanced or recurrent thymomas. LOEHRER et al. reported the results of a multicenter phase I/II study testing the efficacy of combination cisplatin, doxorubicin, and cyclophosphamide (PAC) in 20 evaluable patients with advanced thymomas. There were three complete responders and 11 partial responders, for a total response rate of 14/20 (70%), but it should be noted that radiotherapy was also given in four of the responding patients [44]. A recent update of this experience, excluding patients with limited disease, reported a 50% overall response rate in 30 patients. The median survival time was 38 months, with a 30% 5-year survival. FORNASIERO et al. described 37 patients with advanced stage III and IV thymomas treated with cisplatin, doxorubicin, vincristine, and cyclophosphamide (ADOC). A 43% (16/37) complete response rate and 92% (34/37) overall response rate was seen, with a median overall response duration of 12 months. Seven of the 16 clinical complete responses were confirmed pathologically at the time of subsequent thoracotomy. Unfortunately, despite these impressive response rates, the median survival for the entire group of patients was only 15 months, indicating substantial room for improvement in therapeutic efficiency [45].

The efficacy of currently promising chemotherapeutic regimens require further validation through clinical trials. An ongoing trial conducted by ECOG treats patients with locally advanced disease with PAC combination chemotherapy, followed by definitive radiation therapy. Also, the ECOG and the Southwest Oncology Group are planning a phase II trial utilizing the VIP (VP-16, ifosfamide, cisplatin) regimen for advanced disease [39]. If activity is confirmed in patients with recurrent or metastatic disease, the role of chemotherapy might then be further investigated in the adjuvant management of patients with less advanced disease who nevertheless have a substantial definable risk for local and/or distant failure despite current approaches with radical surgery and radiotherapy. At that point, issues such as sequencing of treatment modalities, as well as the relative importance of each modality, will need to be carefully evaluated to define the optimal therapeutic index [46].

3.4 Conclusions

1. Additional therapy following complete surgical resection is not indicated in patients whose thymomas do not extend beyond the tumor capsule. However, extended follow-up is warranted because of the risk, albeit very low, of late recurrences.
2. We currently recommend postoperative radiotherapy for patients with completely resected stage II thymomas where histologic documentation of disease extension beyond the capsule is seen. Further validation of currently proposed prognostic factors within this population of stage II thymoma patients will allow better selection of those with an excellent chance of cure with surgery alone, versus those who may benefit from adjuvant irradiation.
3. Postoperative radiotherapy should be considered part of comprehensive management in patients with completely resected stage III disease.
4. Incompletely resectable thymomas can be controlled with radical radiotherapy. However, maximal surgical debulking will improve the chances of tumor control. Care must be given to optimize radiation treatment planning to provide adequate tumor coverage as well as to minimize injury to surrounding normal structures.
5. Promising chemotherapeutic regimens have been identified which need to be validated through further evaluation in patients with advanced unresectable, metastatic, and/or recurrent disease. Once established, the role of chemotherapy may be investigated in the management of patients with less advance thymomas, currently treated by surgery and radiotherapy, in whom the risk of both local relapse and distant failure remains substantial.

References

1. Wilkins EW Jr (1995) Thymoma: surgical management. In: Wood DE, Thomas CR Jr (eds), Medical Radiology. Diagnostic Imaging and Radiation Oncology – Mediastinal Tumors. Springer-Verlag, Heidelberg, pp 11–18
2. Marino M, Muller-Hermelink HK (1985) Thymoma and thymic carcinoma. Relation of thymoma epithelial cells to the cortical and medullary differentiation of thymus. Virchows Arch [A] Pathol Anat Histopathol 407: 119–149
3. Verley JM, Hollmann KH (1985) Thymoma. A comparative study of clinical stages, histologic features, and survival in 200 cases. Cancer 55: 1074–1086
4. Pescarmona E, Rendina EA, Venuta F, et al. (1990) Analysis of prognostic factors and clinicopathological staging of thymoma. Ann Thorac Surg 50: 534–538
5. Quintanilla-Martinez L, Wilkins EW Jr, Ferry JA, Harris NL (1993) Thymoma – morphologic subclassification correlates with invasiveness and immunohistologic features: a study of 122 cases. Hum Pathol 24: 958–969
6. Pollack A, El-Nagger AK, Cox JD, Ro JY, Sahin A, Komaki R (1992) Thymoma. The prognostic significance of flow cytometric DNA analysis. Cancer 69: 1702–1709
7. Nakahara K, Ohno K, Hashimoto J, et al. (1988) Thymoma: results with complete resection and adjuvant postoperative irradiation in 141 consecutive patients. J Thorac Cardiovasc Surg 95: 1041–1047
8. Wick MR (1990) Assessing the prognosis of thymomas. Ann Thorac Surg 50: 521–522
9. Maggi G, Casadio C, Cavallo A, Cianci R, Molinatti M, Ruffini E (1991) Thymoma: results of 241 operated cases. Ann Thorac Surg 51: 152–156
10. Wilkins EW Jr, Grillo HC, Scannell JG, Moncure AC, Mathisen DJ (1991) Role of staging in prognosis and management of thymoma. Ann Thorac Surg 51: 888–892
11. Bergh NP, Gatzinsky P, Larsson S, Lundin P, Ridell B (1978) Tumors of the thymus and thymic region I. Clinicopathological studies of thymomas. Ann Thorac Surg 25: 91–98
12. Masaoka A, Monden Y, Nakahara K, Tanioka T (1981) Follow-up study of thymomas with special reference to their clinical stages. Cancer 48: 2485–2492
13. Wilkins EW Jr, Castleman B (1979) Thymoma: a continuing survey at the Massachusetts General Hospital. Ann Thorac Surg 28: 252–256
14. Curran WJ Jr, Kornstein MJ, Brooks JJ, Turrisi AT (1988) Invasive thymoma: the role of mediastinal irradiation following complete or incomplete surgical resection. J Clin Oncol 6: 1722–1727

15. Yamakawa Y, Masaoka A, Hashimoto T, et al. (1991) A tentative tumor-node-metastasis classification of thymoma. Cancer 68: 1983–1987

16. Arakawa A, Yasunaga T, Saitoh Y, et al. (1990) Radiation therapy of invasive thymoma. Int J Radiat Oncol Biol Phys 18: 529–534

17. Jackson MA, Ball DL (1991) Post-operative radiotherapy in invasive thymoma. Radiother Oncol 21: 77–82

18. Batata MA, Martini N, Huvos AG, Aguilar RI, Beattie EJ (1974) Thymomas: clinicopathologic features, therapy, and prognosis. Cancer 34: 389–396

19. Nordstrom DG, Tewfik HH, Latourette HB (1979) Thymoma: therapy and prognosis as related to operative staging. Int J Radiat Oncol Biol Phys 5: 2059–2062

20. Appelqvist P, Kostiainen S, Franssila K, Mattila S, Grohn P (1982) Treatment and prognosis of thymoma: a review of 25 cases. J Surg Oncol 20: 265–268

21. Maggi G, Giaccone G, Donadio M, et al. (1986) Thymomas. A review of 169 cases, with particular reference to results of surgical treatment. Cancer 58: 765–776

22. Haniuda M, Morimoto M, Nishimura H, Kobayashi O, Yamanda T, Iida F (1992) Adjuvant radiotherapy after complete resection of thymoma. Ann Thorac Surg 54: 311–315

23. Pollack A, Komaki R, Cox JD, et al. (1992) Thymoma: treatment and prognosis. Int J Radiat Oncol Biol Phys 23: 1037–1043

24. Etienne T, Deleaval PJ, Spiliopoulos A, Megevand R (1993) Thymoma: prognostic factors. Eur J Cardiothorac Surg 7: 449–452

25. Urgesi A, Monetti U, Rossi G, Ricardi U, Maggi G, Sannazzari GL (1992) Aggressive treatment of intrathoracic recurrences of thymoma. Radiother Oncol 24: 221–225

26. Urgesi A, Monetti U, Rossi G, Ricardi U, Casadio C (1990) Role of radiation therapy in locally advanced thymoma. Radiother Oncol 19: 273–280

27. Chahinian AP, Bhardwaj S, Meyer RJ, Jaffrey IS, Kirschner PA, Holland JF (1981) Treatment of invasive or metastatic thymoma: report of eleven cases. Cancer 47: 1752–1761

28. Marks RD Jr, Wallace KM, Pettit HS (1978) Radiation therapy control of nine patients with malignant thymoma. Cancer 41: 117–119

29. Monden Y, Nakahara K, Iioka S, et al. (1985) Recurrence of thymoma: clinicopathological features, therapy, and prognosis. Ann Thorac Surg 39: 165–169

30. Penn CRH, Hope-Stone HF (1972) The role of radiotherapy in the management of malignant thymoma. Br J Surg 59: 533–539

31. Ariaratnam LS, Kalnicki S, Mincer F, Botstein C (1979) The management of malignant thymoma with radiation therapy. Int J Radiat Oncol Biol Phys 5: 77–80

32. Arriagada R, Bretel JJ, Caillaud JM, et al. (1984) Invasive carcinoma of the thymus. A multicenter retrospective review of 56 cases. Eur J Cancer Clin Oncol 20: 69–74

33. Cohen DJ, Ronnigen LD, Graeber GM, et al. (1984) Management of patients with malignant thymoma. J Thorac Cardiovasc Surg 87: 301–307

34. Kersh CR, Eisert DR, Hazra TA (1985) Malignant thymoma: role of radiation therapy in management. Radiology 156: 207–209

35. Krueger JB, Sagerman RH, King GA (1988) Stage III thymoma: results of postoperative radiation therapy. Radiology 168: 855–858

36. Emami B (1992) Mediastinum and trachea. In: Perez CA, Brady LW (eds) Principles and Practice of Radiation Oncology, 2nd edn. Lippincott, Philadelphia, pp 837–852

37. Uematsu M, Kondo M (1986) A proposal for treatment of invasive thymoma. Cancer 58: 1979–1984

38. Roach M III, Vijayakumar S (1995) The role of three-dimensional conformal radiotherapy in the treatment of mediastinal tumors. In: Wood DE, Thomas CR Jr (eds) Medical Radiology. Diagnostic Imaging and Radiation Oncology-Mediastinal tumors. Springer-Verlag, Heidelberg, pp 117–123

39. Loehrer PJ (1993) Thymomas. Current experience and future directions in therapy. Drugs 45: 477–487

40. Bonomi PD, Finkelstein D, Aisner S, Ettinger D (1993) EST 2582 phase II trial of cisplatin in metastatic or recurrent thymoma. Am J Clin Oncol 16: 342–345

41. Harper PG, Highley M, Rankin E, et al. (1991) Ifosfamide monotherapy demonstrates high activity in malignant thymoma. Proc Am Soc Clin Oncol 10: 300 (abstract #1049)

42. Goldel N, Boning L, Fredrik A, Hozel D, Hartenstein R, Wilmanns W (1989) Chemotherapy of invasive thymoma: a retrospective study of 22 cases. Cancer 63: 1493–1500

43. Hue E, Levine J (1986) Chemotherapy of malignant thymoma: case report and review of the literature. Cancer 57: 1101–1104

44. Loehrer PJ, Perez CA, Roth LM, Greco A, Livingston RB, Einhorn LH (1990) Chemotherapy for advanced thymoma: preliminary results of an intergroup study. Ann Intern Med 113: 520–524

45. Fornasiero A, Daniele O, Ghiotto C, et al. (1991) Chemotherapy for invasive thymoma: a 13-year experience. Cancer 68: 30–33

46. Macchiarini P, Chella A, Ducci F, et al. (1991) Neoadjuvant chemotherapy, surgery, and postoperative radiation therapy for invasive thymoma. Cancer 68: 706–713

4 Mediastinal Lymphomas

STEPHEN H. PETERSDORF

CONTENTS

4.1 Introduction

Malignant lymphoma, including non-Hodgkin's lymphoma and Hodgkin's disease, may involve any organ of the body. Mediastinal involvement may be part of a generalized process or may occur due to a malignant population limited to the mediastinum alone. Hodgkin's disease has long been associated with mediastinal involvement and in recent years, the recognition of high-grade non-Hodgkin's lymphoma limited to the mediastinum has become increasingly common, particularly in young women. Primary mediastinal lymphomas are relatively uncommon in adults, but in children, malignant lymphoma is among the most common of malignant mediastinal neoplasms. The majority of mediastinal lymphomas occur in the anterior or middle mediastinal components. The differential diagnosis of malignant processes in this location includes thymoma, germ cell tumors, and thyroid neoplasms. Lymphomas of the mediastinum usually arise in the lymph nodes, but rarely other tissues such as the thyroid gland may be the site of the primary disease. Mediastinal lymphomas have a wide spectrum of presentation ranging from an incidental finding on routine staging of lymphoma to a localized process associated with bulky adenopathy leading to life-threatening airway obstruction or pericardial tamponade.

4.2 Presentation

Patients with mediastinal lymphoma usually present with symptoms related to mediastinal disease if there is bulky adenopathy. Patients often have symptoms that are a consequence of impingement of the lymphoma on structures within the mediastinum, usually in the anterior or middle compartments. The mediastinum contains several vital structures that may be compressed by or involved with malignant lymphoma, including the trachea, the heart, great vessels including the superior vena cava, the esophagus, and the thyroid gland. Patients with bulky adenopathy are more likely to have compression of one or more of these vital structures, leading to presentation. Superior vena cava syndrome (SVC syndrome) is common in both Hodgkin's disease and mediastinal large cell non-Hodgkin's lymphoma. Presenting symptoms associated with SVC syndrome may include upper extremity and facial edema, venous engorgement, and shortness of breath. The differential diagnosis of patients presenting with SVC syndrome includes lymphoma, thymoma, lung cancer, germ cell tumor, and breast cancer. Other presenting complaints associated with mediastinal lymphoma may include shortness of breath due to direct tracheal compression, hoarseness due to recurrent laryngeal nerve involvement, dysphagia due to esophageal compression, and chest pain due to pericardial, pleural, or chest wall invasion. Fevers, night sweats, and weight loss are common systemic complaints that are frequently seen in patients with Hodgkin's disease. Patients may have evidence of supraclavicular adenopathy or of diffuse adenopathy. Pleural and pericardial effusion may also be present. Furthermore, patients with a histologically high-grade tumor (i.e., lymphoblastic lymphoma) may

STEPHEN H. PETERSDORF, M.D., Assistant Professor, Division of Medical Oncology, RC-08, University of Washington, Seattle, WA 98195, USA present with rapid onset of symptoms over a period of hours to days as the tumor may reach a critical mass within a short period.

4.3 Diagnosis

In order to determine an appropriate treatment plan, the extent of the lymphoma as well as the histologic subtype of the lymphoma needs to be determined. Initial evaluation typically includes a chest roentgenogram and a computed tomography (CT) scan of the chest, abdomen, and pelvis. CT examination may distinguish normal structures from abnormal structures as well as determine the extent and location of mediastinal adenopathy. Magnetic resonance imaging (MRI) scans also may be used to evaluate the mediastinum, particularly in those patients who cannot receive iodinated contrast. MRI is also superior to CT imaging when defining lesions in the posterior mediastinum that may extend into the spinal canal. However, CT scans remain superior to determine pathologic calcification as well as spatial planes [1]. Additional staging studies to determine the extent of the disease will be described below.

Once the extent of mediastinal involvement has been determined, an attempt at histologic diagnosis should be made. If there is peripheral adenopathy, the peripheral lymph node should be resected before more invasive techniques are pursued. However, in many instances of mediastinal lymphoma, the disease is localized to the mediastinum and more invasive procedures are required. Transthoracic fine-needle aspiration (TFNA) or a cutting needle biopsy usually can be performed with CT, fluoroscopic, or ultrasound guidance for most tissues within the mediastinum. The contraindications to these procedures include the presence of a hydatid cyst, a bleeding disorder, a suspected vascular lesion, advanced emphysema, previous pneumonectomy, and pulmonary hypertension. While a TFNA or cutting needle biopsy may differentiate between a nonlymphomatous process and a lymphoma, the small sample usually precludes the accurate evaluation of the type of lymphoma. Since the treatment depends on distinguishing Hodgkin's disease from non-Hodgkin's disease as well as the subtypes of non-Hodgkin's lymphoma, a needle biopsy is usually not sufficient to determine a treatment plan and a TFNA is never adequate to determine the true malignant histology. If there is a high index of suspicion for the mediastinal mass being due to a lymphoma, a

more invasive diagnostic procedure must be pursued to obtain adequate tissue.

Mediastinoscopy, anterior mediastinotomy, or even a median sternotomy or thoracotomy may be required to obtain adequate tissue. Mediastinoscopy has historically been the procedure of choice as it is a safe, well-tolerated procedure with a high likelihood of obtaining a diagnosis with minimal morbidity [2]. A recent trial by ELIA et al. compared cervical mediastinoscopy with anterior mediastinotomy for the diagnosis of mediastinal lymphoma [3]. All 95 patients on this trial underwent a screening TFNA to rule out a carcinoma or infection, and while all of these patients were ultimately determined to have lymphoma, this diagnosis was documented in only 12 patients who underwent TFNA. Patients were then divided into four groups. Twenty-two patients with an anterior mediastinal mass underwent anterior mediastinoscopy, 19 with a middle mediastinal mass underwent cervical mediastinoscopy, and the remaining 54 patients were randomized to either mediastinoscopy or anterior mediastinotomy. The overall diagnostic accuracy was 80.43% for cervical mediastinoscopy and 95.91% for anterior mediastinotomy. This difference was statistically significant ($P < 0.025$). Nine patients who underwent a cervical mediastinoscopy required a median sternotomy or thoracotomy to obtain the diagnosis whereas two patients who underwent a anterior mediastinotomy required a second procedure. Both procedures appear to have a high likelihood of success in obtaining the diagnosis. Anterior mediastinotomy may be slightly better, especially for anterior mediastinal lesions, although this procedure may be associated with slightly more surgical trauma.

Patients with bulky mediastinal mass may occasionally present with airway obstruction and may require intubation and mechanical ventilation. However, an attempt to make a histologic diagnosis should be pursued wherever it is safe and feasible. A biopsy in this situation may occasionally be too hazardous and so emergent radiotherapy is often initiated prior to making a diagnosis. However, initiation of radiotherapy may preclude accurate histologic diagnosis which may compromise eventual curative therapy. Prompt medical therapy is another approach that may shrink the mass sufficiently for a safe biopsy without disrupting the histology. Patients may receive a single standard parenteral dose of an alkylating agent or a dose of corticosteroids to shrink the tumor without disrupting the malignant architecture, after which a biopsy may be performed promptly [4]. This approach appears to be less likely to alter the histology of the tumor for analysis and would not compromise future care.

Once the biopsy is obtained, the sample should be processed to determine the nature of the lymphoma. Whenever lymphoma is suspected, a portion of the biopsy should be snap frozen in order to perform cell surface marker studies as well as immunoglobulin gene rearrangement studies or T-cell receptor studies. In addition to routine histologic studies, hematopathologic studies can distinguish Hodgkin's disease from non-Hodgkin's lymphoma and can determine B-cell and T-cell neoplasms. The three most common mediastinal lymphomas that will be discussed further each have distinctive immunophenotyping [5]. Hodgkin's disease typically is positive for CD15 and CD30. Large cell lymphoma of the mediastinum, which is a B-cell process, is usually positive for CD45 as well as the B-cell lineage markers, including CD19, CD20, and CD22. CD30 and k/λ surface proteins also may be positive in large-cell lymphoma. Lymphoblastic lymphoma is a T-cell malignancy that commonly affects children and young adults. The immunophenotypic markers for this lymphoma reflect this cell of origin, with positive markers including CD45, TdT, CD1, and the pan-T-cell markers (CD2, CD3, CD5, CD7, CD43, and CD45RO). Many of these antibodies are effective only on fresh frozen tissue and so all biopsies should be processed to have both frozen and paraffin-embedded tissue available for study.

4.4 Evaluation and Staging

Lymphoma may involve the mediastinum alone or may be part of a generalized process. Hodgkin's disease is more likely to have involvement of the mediastinum than is non-Hodgkin's lymphoma: while 20% of patients with non-Hodgkin's lymphoma have mediastinal involvement at presentation, 50% of patients with Hodgkin's disease have such involvement. Women account for 70% of Hodgkin's disease patients with mediastinal involvement [4]. Patients with non-Hodgkin's lymphoma may have either a T-cell lymphoma or a B-cell phenotype. Mediastinal B-cell lymphomas are thought to be derived from mediastinal lymph nodes whereas T-cell neoplasms probably arise from the thymic tissues [6]. While disseminated lymphomas may involve the mediastinum, there are two distinct types

of non-Hodgkin's lymphoma that may be localized to the mediastinum: mediastinal large cell lymphoma and lymphoblastic lymphoma.

As part of the evaluation of a patient with a mediastinal mass, initial staging procedures are standard for every patient with lymphoma. These studies include a detailed history with attention to shortness of breath, fever (greater than 101 °F), night sweats, and weight loss. Physical examination should include close evaluation of the lymph nodes, liver, and spleen. Laboratory evaluation should include a complete blood count with differential, renal function evaluation, liver function tests including lactate dehydrogenase (LDH) determination, determination of the uric acid level, and an arterial blood gas measurement if there is any evidence of respiratory compromise. The LDH level is an important prognostic factor as it is frequently elevated in high-grade lymphomas such as Burkitt's lymphoma, diffuse large cell lymphoma, and lymphoblastic lymphoma. The LDH level also can be followed as the disease is treated as the level will decrease as the patient responds. Additional staging studies are performed for both Hodgkin's disease and non-Hodgkin's lymphoma to determine the extent of disease, which, particularly for Hodgkin's disease, is critical when constructing the therapeutic plan and establishing the prognosis. Typical staging studies would include CT scan of the chest, abdomen, and pelvis, lymphangiography, and bone marrow examination. Other studies such as a bone scan or gallium scan may be performed where clinically appropriate. The Ann Arbor staging system is standard for Hodgkin's disease and is often applied when describing the stage of disease in patients with non-Hodgkin's lymphoma (Table 4.1).

Table 4.1. Ann Arbor staging system for lymphoma[a]

Stage I	Involvement of a single lymph node region or a single extralymphatic organ or site
Stage II	Involvement of two or more lymph node regions on the same side of the diaphragm or localized to an extralymphatic organ or site by extension
Stage III	Involvement of lymph node regions on both sides of the diaphragm or localized involvement of an extralymphatic site (III_e) or spleen (III_s) or both (III_{se})
Stage IV	Diffuse or disseminated involvement of one or more extralymphatic organs with or without associated nodal involvement

[a] For all stages, A = asymptomatic, B = fever > 101 °F, night sweats, and weight loss greater than 10% of body weight, E = extranodal site, S = spleen

Once the histology is determined and the stage defined, appropriate therapy can be instituted. The most common types of lymphoma that have a mediastinal component are Hodgkin's disease, lymphoblastic lymphoma, and mediastinal B-cell lymphoma. Each of these will be discussed below.

4.5 Evaluation and Treatment of Mediastinal Lymphoma

4.5.1 Hodgkin's Disease

Hodgkin's disease (HD) is the most common primary lymphoma of the mediastinum and has a predilection to affect young women. HD is usually characterized by an orderly progression of lymph node involvement so that patients with mediastinal HD may present with cervical or supraclavicular lymphadenopathy. Mediastinal involvement with HD is more common in young women, who often present with rapid onset of symptoms due to bulky mediastinal adenopathy. These patients may have evidence of SVC syndrome as well as systemic complaints such as fever, night sweats, and weight loss.

There are four histologic subtypes of HD (Table 4.2). Patients with lymphocyte-predominant and nodular sclerosing HD generally have a better prognosis; furthermore, these subtypes typically present with early-stage disease. Patients with mixed cellularity or lymphocyte-depleted HD are more likely to present with advanced disease. The majority of patients with mediastinal HD have the nodular sclerosing subtype.

The treatment of HD is dictated less by the histologic subtype than by the extent of tumor. All histologic subtypes are treated in a similar manner and so staging of the disease is essential to determine appropriate therapy. Staging procedures that may be used to determine whether the patient has stage II, III, or IV disease include:

1. Chest, abdomen, and pelvic CT scan
2. Lymphangiography
3. Bilateral bone marrow biopsy

4. Gallium scan
5. Exploratory laparotomy with splenectomy and liver biopsy

The purpose of staging is to determine whether patients may be treated with radiotherapy alone. The latter is particularly appropriate for early-stage, asymptomatic HD, where up to 95% of patients with pathologically staged IA or IIA HD and low-volume mediastinal adenopathy may be cured when treated with appropriate mantle radiotherapy [7]. Patients who are symptomatic with B symptoms are less likely to be cured, with 75% of these patients achieving long-term disease-free survival with radiotherapy alone [8]. Consequently, if a patient is being considered for radiotherapy alone and all staging studies, including CT scans, lymphangiography, and the bone marrow examination, are negative, exploratory laparotomy should be considered. Clinical trials are currently underway to determine whether patients with stage IA and IIA low-volume disease can be treated with radiotherapy alone without undergoing exploratory laparotomy.

Patients with bulky mediastinal adenopathy at any stage of disease have a high rate of relapse when treated with radiotherapy or chemotherapy alone. Bulky adenopathy is defined as adenopathy greater than one-third of the chest diameter on an upright anteroposterior chest radiograph. The Stanford group has reported a 45% disease-free survival for those patients with stage I or II disease and large mediastinal adenopathy treated with radiotherapy alone [9]. Other studies have demonstrated a similar poor prognosis for these patients treated with radiotherapy alone [10]. Patients treated with chemotherapy alone have a similar poor prognosis. Combined modality therapy with radiotherapy and chemotherapy appears to provide a marked improvement in outcome for those patients with large mediastinal adenopathy. While those patients who relapse after treatment with radiotherapy alone may be salvaged with chemotherapy, the overall survival is still inferior to that in patients treated with initial combined modality therapy [11].

Combined modality therapy eliminates the need for staging laparotomy since patients receive systemic chemotherapy. Different approaches to combined modality therapy have been attempted with different sequences of treatment as well as different chemotherapeutic regimens. Combined modality therapy has been administered in different orders, including chemotherapy–radiotherapy, radiotherapy–chemotherapy, or the "sandwich technique" where half the chemotherapy is delivered prior to radio-

Table 4.2. Histologic subtypes of HD

Subtype	Frequency
Lymphocyte-predominant	5%–15%
Nodular sclerosing	50%–70%
Mixed cellularity	20%–40%
Lymphocyte-depleted	5%–10%

therapy and the remainder is delivered at the conclusion of radiotherapy. BEHAR et al. from the Stanford group recently reported 48 patients with bulky mediastinal adenopathy treated between 1980 and 1988 [12]. Only the first ten patients underwent exploratory laparotomy. Radiotherapy was administered to 40 Gy, with a shrinking field technique used after 15–20 Gy had been delivered. Chemotherapy consisted of either MOPP (nitrogen mustard, vincristine, procarbazine, and prednisone), ABVD (Adriamycin, bleomycin, vinblastine, and decarbazine), or pAVE (melphelan, vinblastine, and procarbazine). The actuarial survival and freedom from relapse were 84% and 89% at 9 years. Other centers have produced similar results for combined modality therapy. Combined modality therapy with involved field radiotherapy is also appropriate for those patients with stage III or stage IV disease with large mediastinal adenopathy [10].

While the standard of treatment for patients with large mediastinal adenopathy is combined modality therapy with chemotherapy and radiotherapy, further clinical trials are needed to address several issues regarding combined modality therapy. The questions to be answered include:

1. Does the order of the chemotherapy/radiotherapy sequence affect patient outcome?
2. What chemotherapy regimen should be used, i.e., is MOPP, MOPP/ABVD, or ABVD the preferred regimen? While MOPP/ABVD or ABVD alone appeared superior in a recent CALGB trial for advanced stage HD, would MOPP be preferable to an ABVD regimen in combined modality treatment where the cardiac (Adriamycin) and pulmonary (bleomycin) toxicities of ABVD may be exacerbated by radiotherapy to the thorax. Conversely, is the combination of MOPP and radiotherapy associated with an increased risk of secondary malignancies, e.g., breast cancer in women.
3. Can the dose of either the chemotherapy or the radiotherapy be reduced when both modalities are used together?

4.5.1.1 Complications Associated with Treatment of Mediastinal Hodgkin's Disease

While a very high proportion of patients with HD and mediastinal adenopathy are cured, treatment-related complications have been observed in a significant proportion of patients. Most of these treatment-related sequelae are due to the effects of radiation therapy in the field. These complications include an increased risk of secondary malignancies, particularly breast cancer. Now that women who were cured of their HD are living longer, there appears to be an increased risk of breast cancer in those women treated with mantle radiotherapy. The risk appears greatest in those women who are under the age of 15 (relative risk 136) at the time of treatment, but all women under the age of 30 appear to be at increased risk. The risk is greater for those women who have also received chemotherapy with MOPP. In the study by HANCOCK et al. [13], the relative risk for all women treated with mantle radiotherapy to die of breast cancer when compared to a normal population was calculated to be 5.1. Women who have received mantle radiotherapy clearly need close observation, including mammograms, to detect the possible occurrence of breast cancer.

Several other complications may occur as a result of mantle radiotherapy. Acute pericarditis with an effusion occurs in 20%–50% of patients [14]. Chronic cardiac disease including chronic constrictive pericarditis and an increased risk of coronary artery disease may also occur after radiotherapy [15]. Since, despite all best efforts, normal lung is invariably part of the radiation field, acute radiation fibrosis will occur in up to 20% of patients with HD. A minority of these patients proceed to develop pulmonary fibrosis. Finally, since the thyroid gland is involved in the mantle field, thyroid dysfunction ranging from clinical hypothyroidism to Graves' disease or malignant thyroid nodules occurs in up to two-thirds of patients [16]. Hypothyroidism may be a late phenomenon occurring more than 5 years after therapy.

4.5.1.2 Residual Mass After Treatment

At the completion of therapy for HD with large mediastinal adenopathy, a residual mass often remains on chest radiograph or CT scan. This is particularly common in those patients with nodular sclerosing HD [17]. The clinical issue is whether this mass represents residual disease or fibrosis. Several approaches have been taken to resolve this dilemma. The most conservative approach is to monitor the mass by serial CT scans obtained every 4–12 weeks for a year. If there is no change in the mass, the residual mass probably represents fibrosis. Any increase in size of the mass is suspicious for tumor and should prompt a biopsy of the mass. Gallium scanning may be a useful diagnostic test; a negative gallium scan, particularly in the setting of a positive pretreatment scan, is useful to distinguish fibrosis from a residual mass [18]. MRI has also been reported to be a useful technique to distinguish fibrosis from residual disease. Usually, either serial radiologic evaluation with CT scans or gallium scanning can provide sufficient information to indicate whether the mass is suspicious for residual tumor.

4.5.2 Non-Hodgkin's Lymphoma

Mediastinal involvement with non-Hodgkin's lymphoma (NHL) is much more likely to be part of a generalized process than is seen with Hodgkin's disease. NHL is usually classified as either nodular or diffuse, and is further classified by the size and malignant appearance of the cells. There are ten subtypes of NHL in the working formulation and there are several other histologic variations that are not described in the working formulation. The histologic subtypes are classified in terms of their appearance as well as their behavior so that lymphomas are classified as low, intermediate, or high grade. Any of the histologic subtypes may involve the mediastinum but primary mediastinal lymphoma is most likely to be an intermediate- or high-grade process. Of all patients with NHL, approximately 20% will have mediastinal involvement at the time of initial evaluation, and fewer than a third of these patients will have disease limited to the mediastinum [19]. Follicular or low-grade lymphomas rarely present with bulky adenopathy or disease limited to the mediastinum. Patients with mediastinal adenopathy as part of a generalized process who do not have bulk disease should be treated as appropriate for the subtype of lymphoma. There are two unique types of NHL that are more likely to present with adenopathy limited to the mediastinum. Patients with primary mediastinal lymphoma, which often presents with bulky adenopathy, typically have either T-cell lymphoblastic lymphoma or a B-cell diffuse large cell or immunoblastic lymphoma.

The staging studies appropriate for patients with these or any of the other NHLs include the same laboratory studies (including LDH determination) as would be obtained for the patient with Hodgkin's disease, CT scans of the chest, abdomen, and pelvis, and bilateral bone marrow biopsies; for patients with high-grade lymphomas with marrow involvement or patients with lymphoblastic lymphoma, lumbar puncture with CSF examination should also be performed. Lymphangiography and exploratory laparotomy are rarely performed in the staging evaluation of patients with NHL as most patients receive systemic chemotherapy.

4.5.2.1 Lymphoblastic Lymphoma

T-cell lymphoblastic lymphoma is a high-grade lymphoma that represents the lymphomatous version of acute lymphoblastic leukemia (ALL). This entity is typically found in children or young adults. There is a 2:1 ratio of males to females with this disease. T-cell lymphoblastic lymphoma accounts for less than 5% of adult lymphomas but accounts for one-third to two-thirds of childhood lymphomas [20]. Between 75% and 80% of patients will present with an anterior mediastinal tumor mass which may be associated with SVC syndrome, pleural effusion, or pericardial effusion [21]. The cytology from the pleural and pericardial fluid is rarely positive. There is considerable overlap with T-cell ALL as lymphoblastic lymphoma may have bone marrow involvement, although there is less likely to be cytopenia or a marked increase in circulating immature blast cells in lymphoblastic lymphoma.

The cell of origin for T-cell lymphoblastic lymphoma is probably the immature T cell although the cells seen in T-cell ALL are derived from a more primitive T-cell precursor. The cells are TdT (terminal deoxytransferase) positive, which is pathognomic of lymphoblastic lymphoma. Most patients present with a mediastinal mass but adenopathy in other sites may be limited. However, bone marrow and central nervous system involvement is common in T-cell lymphoblastic lymphoma. All patients with lymphoblastic lymphoma need examination of the CSF and subsequent treatment directed to the CNS with intrathecal chemotherapy ± craniospinal radiotherapy. Lymphoblastic lymphoma is nearly always a T-cell process in children and is a T-cell process in 80%–90% of adults. B-cell lymphoblastic lymphoma is relatively rare; it is not associated with a mediastinal mass but often has marrow involvement and is characterized by a very aggressive course.

If patients with lymphoblastic lymphoma are treated with a regimen intended for other lymphomas, such as CHOP (cyclophosphamide, hydroxydaunomycin, Oncovin, and prednisone), the prognosis is quite poor. However, significant improvement in therapy has been made by treating this disease in a manner similar to childhood acute lymphoblastic leukemia. Most regimens utilize an intensive anthracycline-based induction regimen with consolidation, CNS prophylaxis with intrathecal chemotherapy with or without cranial radiotherapy, and maintenance therapy. COLEMAN et al. have reported treatment results in 44 patients treated with a four-phase protocol with induction, CNS prophylaxis, consolidation with four cycles of the induction therapy, and maintenance therapy with oral methotrexate and 6-mercaptopurine for 1 year. The overall complete response rate was 95%, with a 3-year freedom from relapse of 58% [21]. Other investigators have demonstrated similar results, with a high rate of complete response, with this type of treatment approach [22]. While these patients often present with bulky mediastinal disease, the use of mediastinal radiotherapy is uncommon as most patients achieve a complete response with chemotherapy. There has been no proven benefit from the addition of mediastinal radiotherapy in this setting. Patients at high risk of relapse appear to be those who present with an LDH > 300 or those who present with stage IV disease [23]. The presence of bulky adenopathy, bone marrow, or CSF involvement does not appear to confer a worse prognosis. For those patients who achieve a remission but are at high risk of relapse, or those who do eventually relapse, more intensive treatments such as bone marrow transplantation should be considered.

4.5.3 Mediastinal Large Cell Lymphoma

Large cell and immunoblastic lymphoma is the most common subtype of primary non-Hodgkin's lymphoma of the mediastinum in adults. This lymphoma appears to be a distinct clinical entity given the differences in the behavior and natural history of diffuse large cell lymphoma in other locations [24]. Patients with this disease often have their disease limited to the thorax at presentation. While the lymphoma appears to originate from the mediastinum, extension beyond the mediastinal lymph nodes into the pleura, pericardium, and lung does occur, with all of the complications of similar large mediastinal masses. Several series have now been published reviewing mediastinal large cell lymphoma. In general, these lymphomas are characterized by bulky adenopathy (> 10 cm) and are limited to the thorax with pleural and pericardial effusions [25]. Compared with large cell and immunoblastic lymphoma in other sites of the body, mediastinal large cell lymphoma is much less likely to be disseminated. The largest review of this entity by KIRN et al. analyzed 57 patients. The median age of patients

at diagnosis was 30; this is similar to other published studies [26] and is younger than the typical patient population with large cell and immunoblastic lymphoma. While there was a slight male predominance in this study, most studies have suggested that females with this diagnosis outnumber men by a 2:1 ratio.

Patients tend to present rather acutely due to locally bulky and growing mediastinal mass. The disease is usually limited to the chest but may be associated with unusual sites of spread, including an increased frequency of renal involvement. The histologic features of this lymphoma are frequently atypical. Mediastinal large cell lymphoma is almost invariably a B-cell process, although 6 of 30 patients analyzed by Kirn had a T-cell phenotype. The histology is notable for large clear cells and sclerosis is frequently present. All 57 patients in Kirn's study had evidence of sclerosis but the amount of sclerosis was variable. In fact, several investigators, including TODESCHINI and co-workers, have noted the extensive sclerosis often found in mediastinal large cell lymphoma [27]. However, the amount of sclerosis does not appear to affect the prognosis [26]. Evaluation of gene rearrangements in these patients raises the possibility of a relationship to Burkitt's lymphoma. SCARPA et al. evaluated six patients with this entity for the presence of c-*myc* and bcl-2, and for evidence of the Epstein-Barr virus (EBV) DNA sequences in the genome of these neoplastic populations. None of the patients had evidence of bcl-2 rearrangement or the EBV genome. There was evidence of alteration of c-*myc* in three of the patients; two of these patients had rearrangements similar to that seen in endemic Burkitt's lymphoma and the third had a rearrangement similar to that seen in spontaneous Burkitt's lymphoma [28].

The prognosis associated with the diagnosis of mediastinal large cell lymphoma has historically been thought to be poor; however, recent data suggest that the prognosis may not be so dismal. An early series by LICHTENSTEIN et al. noted a 20% long-term disease-free survival [24]. Newer series demonstrate improved survival (Table 4.3) that is similar to diffuse large cell lymphoma presenting in other locations.

All patients were treated with an anthracycline-based regimen. While none of the patients in the Todeschini study obtained a complete remission with CHOP and required more intensive regimens, patients in the other studies obtained complete responses with CHOP as well as more intensive regimens such as MACOP-B or M-BACOD. The

Table 4.3. Treatment results in patients with large cell mediastinal lymphoma

Study	No. of patients	% bulk disease	CR rate	5-year disease-free survival
JACOBSON et al. [25]	30	65%	80%	59%
TODESCHINI et al. [27]	21	76%	62%	57%
KIRN et al. [26]	57	76%	53%	45%

optimal chemotherapy regimen for mediastinal large cell lymphoma has not been determined, but CHOP has not been proven to be inferior to more intensive regimens in the treatment of diffuse large cell lymphoma in other locations [29]. All of these series suggest that the response to treatment with Adriamycin-containing regimens is similar to that in patients with large cell lymphoma in other sites. Combined modality therapy with mediastinal radiotherapy has also been sporadically employed in all of these studies. Twenty patients in the Kirn study received radiotherapy; there was a decreased overall relapse rate in the radiotherapy group that did not achieve statistical significance. The role of radiotherapy, even in patients with bulky mediastinal adenopathy at presentation, remains unclear. Patients in the Kirn series who received radiotherapy for a positive posttreatment gallium scan did not benefit from the addition of radiotherapy.

Prognostic features have been analyzed in each of the aforementioned series. In the Jacobson review, the presence of bulk disease was associated with an increased risk of relapse. In the larger series of Kirn, the presence of pleural or pericardial effusion was the single most significant risk factor for relapse, and the presence of effusion did not correlate with the presence of bulk disease. Almost all patients with pleural effusion relapsed. Bulky mediastinal adenopathy was a risk factor if an effusion was not present. Other factors associated with an increased risk of relapse include the presence of two or more extranodal sites of disease at presentation, residual mass at the conclusion of chemotherapy, the presence of a positive gallium-67 scan at the conclusion of chemotherapy, or an LDH level three times normal at presentation. Thus, patients who present with a pleural effusion or involvement at two or more extranodal sites at diagnosis should be considered for more intensive therapy than is standard owing to the high likelihood of relapse.

4.6 Summary

The mediastinum is a common site for the development of lymphoma in children and young adults. The most notable mediastinal lymphomas – Hodgkin's disease, lymphoblastic lymphoma, and mediastinal large cell lymphoma – present with bulky adenopathy and symptoms related to this adenopathy. These lymphomas are typically aggressive but are curable with chemotherapy and, when clinically indicated, radiotherapy. Careful pathologic diagnosis as well as staging is critical to a successful outcome. Further recognition of the unique behavior of mediastinal Hodgkin's disease with large mediastinal adenopathy, lymphoblastic lymphoma, and mediastinal large cell lymphoma should lead to further clinical investigation regarding the optimal management of patients with these malignancies.

References

1. Hoffman O, Gillespie D, Aughenbaugh G, Brown L (1993) Primary mediastinal neoplasms (other than thymoma). Mayo Clin Proc 68: 880–891
2. Ricci C, Rendina E, Venuta F, et al. (1990) Surgical approach to isolated mediastinal lymphoma. J Thorac Cardiovasc Surg 99: 691–695
3. Elia S, Cecere C, Giampaglia F, Ferrante G (1992) Mediastinoscopy vs. anterior mediastinotomy in the diagnosis of mediastinal lymphoma: a randomized trial. Eur J Cardiothorac Surg 6: 361–365
4. Dutcher J, Wiernik P (1989) Lymphomas involving the mediastinum and lungs. In: Roth J, Ruckdeschul J, Weisenburger T (eds) Thoracic oncology, 2nd edn. Saunders, Philadelphia, pp 448–465
5. Strickler J, Kurtin P (1991) Mediastinal lymphoma. Semin Diagn Pathol 8: 2–13
6. Kaplan J, Mastrangelo R, Peterson W Jr (1974) Childhood lymphoblastic lymphoma, a cancer of thymus derived lymphocytes. Cancer Res 34: 521–525
7. Rosenberg S, Kaplan H (1985) The evolution and summary results of the Stanford randomized clinical trials of the management of Hodgkin's disease: 1962–1984. Int J Radiat Oncol Biol Phys 11(2): 5–22

8. Crnkovich M, Hoppe R, Rosenberg S (1986) Stage IIB Hodgkin's disease: the Stanford experience. J Clin Oncol 4: 472–479

9. Hoppe R, Coleman C, Cox R, et al. (1982) The management of stage I–II Hodgkin's disease with irradiation alone or combined modality therapy. The Stanford experience. Blood 59: 455–465

10. Leslie N, Mauch P, Hellman S (1985) Stage IA to IIB supradiaphragmatic Hodgkin's disease. Cancer 55: 2072–2078

11. Mauch P, Hellman S (1980) Supradiaphramatic Hodgkin's disease: is there a role for MOPP chemotherapy in patients with bulky mediastinal disease? Int J Radiat Oncol Biol Phys 6: 809–813

12. Behar R, Horning S, Hoppe R (1993) Hodgkin's disease with bulky mediastinal involvement: effective management with combined modality therapy. Int J Radiat Oncol Biol Phys 25: 771–776

13. Hancock S, Tucker M, Hoppe R (1993) Breast cancer after treatment of Hodgkin's disease. J Natl Cancer Inst 85: 25–31

14. Ruckdeschel J, Chang P, Martin R, et al. (1975) Radiation related pericardial effusions in patients with Hodgkin's disease. Medicine (Baltimore) 54: 245–259

15. Boivin J, Hutchison G (1982) Coronary heart disease mortality after irradiation for Hodgkin's disease. Cancer 49: 2470–2475

16. Hancock S, Cox R, McDougall I (1991) Thyroid diseases after Hodgkin's disease. N Engl J Med 325: 599–605

17. Jochelson M, Mauch P, Balikian J, et al. (1985) The significance of the residual mediastinal mass in treated Hodgkin's disease. J Clin Oncol 3: 637–640

18. Gasparini M, Balzarini L, Castellani M, et al. (1993) Current role of gallium scan and magnetic resonance imaging in the management of mediastinal Hodgkin lymphoma. Cancer 72: 577–582

19. Jones S, Fuks Z, Bull M, et al. (1973) Non-Hodgkin's lymphomas. IV. Clinicopathologic correlation in 405 cases. Cancer 31: 806–823

20. Rosenberg SA (1982) The non-Hodgkin's lymphoma pathologic classification project. The National Cancer Institute sponsored study of classifications of non-Hodgkin's lymphomas. Cancer 49: 2112–2135

21. Coleman C, Picozzi V Jr, Cox R, et al. (1986) Treatment of lymphoblastic lymphoma in adults. J Clin Oncol 4: 1628–1637

22. Weinstein H, Cassady J, Levey R (1983) Long term results of the APO protocol (vincristine, doxorubicin (Adriamycin) and prednisone) for treatment of mediastinal lymphoblastic lymphoma. J Clin Oncol 1: 537–541

23. Picozzi V Jr, Coleman C (1990) Lymphoblastic Lymphoma. Semin Oncol 17: 96–103

24. Lichtenstein A, Levine A, Taylor C, et al. (1980) Primary mediastinal lymphoma in adults. Am J Med 68: 509–514

25. Jacobson J, Aisenberg A, Lamarre L, et al. (1988) Mediastinal large cell lymphoma: an uncommon subset of adult lymphoma cureable with combined modality therapy. Cancer 62: 1893–1897

26. Kirn D, Mauch P, Shaffer K, et al. (1993) Large-cell and immunoblastic lymphoma of the mediastinum: prognostic features and treatment outcome in 57 patients. J Clin Oncol 11: 1336–1343

27. Todeschini G, Ambrosetti A, Meneghini V, et al. (1990) Mediastinal large-B-cell lymphoma with sclerosis: a clinical study of 21 patients. J Clin Oncol 8: 804–808

28. Scarpa A, Borgato L, Chilosi M, et al. (1991) Evidence of c-*myc* gene abnormalities in mediastinal large B-cell lymphoma of young adult age. Blood 78: 780–788

29. Fisher R, Gaynor E, Dahlberg S, et al. (1993) Comparison of a standard regimen (CHOP) with three intensive chemotherapy regimens for advanced non-Hodgkin's lymphoma. N Engl J Med 329: 1002–1006

5 Benign Mediastinal Germ Cell Tumors

Mark S. Allen

CONTENTS

5.1 Introduction

Benign germ cell tumors of the mediastinum are commonly referred to as teratomas. Teratomas are defined as tumors or neoplasms that are composed of tissue that is foreign to the organ or anatomic site in which they arise [1]. The additional requirement that all three germ layers, ectoderm, mesoderm, and endoderm, be present is often included in a definition of a teratoma. However, this is not an absolute requirement since with incomplete differentiation, one or two of the layers may be missing.

A variety of nomenclature has been used to describe benign germ cell tumors of the mediastinum. The simplest is to use the term "teratoma." The term "teratoma" comes from the Greek *teratos*, meaning monster, which reflects the often bizarre appearance of these tumors. The terms "teratoblastoma," "teratoid tumor," and "embryoma" are all misleading and should not be used. Similarly, the terms "bidermoma" and "tridermoma," which try to specify the number of germ layers present, are cumbersome and are, fortunately, rarely used today. The term "dermoid cyst" is commonly used and refers to the cystic appearance of the tumor.

About 10%–20% of mediastinal masses will be germ cell tumors, depending on the age group studied [2]. Mediastinal germ cell tumors account for only 3%–5% of all germ cell tumors, but the mediastinum is the most common extragonadal site for a germ cell tumor to arise. The different types of germ cell tumors that occur in the mediastinum include benign teratoma, seminoma (dysgerminoma), embryonal cell carcinoma, endodermal sinus tumor (yolk sac tumor), choriocarcinoma, and mixed cell tumors [3]. Unlike germ cell tumors of the testes, which are usually malignant, germ cell tumors in the mediastinum are three to four times more likely to be benign [4]. Benign teratomas can be further classified as mature or immature and solid or cystic.

5.2 Incidence and Epidemiology

In a review from the Mayo Clinic, Lewis et al. found that 8% of mediastinal tumors are benign teratomas [5]. In patients less than 16 years old, the incidence of benign germ cell tumors is second only to neurogenic tumors in the mediastinum [6]. The sex distribution of benign teratomas is about equal, but most malignant germ cell tumors in the mediastinum are in males. The median age when the tumor is diagnosed is 28 years, but these tumors have occurred in patients from 1 month of age to 73 years old.

There are a few predisposing factors that are associated with the development of a mediastinal germ cell tumor. Patients with Klinefelter's syndrome have a higher risk of developing a germ cell tumor [7]. There is a case report of non-twin brothers who both developed teratomatous tumors, but there is no firm evidence that teratomas are genetically transmitted.

Most of the tumors arise in the anterosuperior portion of the mediastinum; only 3% arise in the posterior mediastinum [8]. Teratomas can occur in almost any area in the body, but the mediastinum is the most common site. Other sites where teratomas have been reported include the sacrococcygeal region, intrapericardium, the orbit, the neck, liver, stomach, and retroperitoneum.

Mark S. Allen, M.D., Assistant Professor of Surgery, Section of General Thoracic Surgery, Mayo Clinic, 200 First Street S.W., Rochester, MN 55905, USA

5.3 Theories of Origin

There are a variety of theories that attempt to explain the origin of a mediastinal teratoma. The reader is referred to GONZALEZ-CRUSSI for a complete discussion of these theories [9]. In brief, the most accepted theory is that a teratoma arises from primordial germ cells that were caught in the mediastinum during embryologic development. In the ovum, cells differentiate into three distinct lines: the somatic line, which goes on to make up the mesoderm, ectoderm, and endoderm, the extraembryonic line, which forms the yolk sac and trophoblast, and the germ cell line, which contains totipotential cells that give rise to the sex cells. As indicated above, it is from germ cells somehow arrested in their migration to the gonads that mediastinal teratomas are thought to originate. Other theories state that the cell of origin for a teratoma differs depending on the site of origin, or that teratomas are a form of maldeveloped conjoined twins.

5.4 Clinical Presentation

The typical patient with a teratoma of mediastinum is discovered by a routine chest roentgenogram (Fig. 5.1). This has only recently been true. In the Mayo series, 23% of the patients were asymptomatic between 1930 and 1953, whereas 53% of the patients were asymptomatic in the period from 1953 to 1981 [5]. This may reflect the increased use of chest roentgenograms as a screening tool.

When symptoms are present, they are from local growth of the mass and compressive symptoms. Chest pain, dyspnea, and cough are the most common complaints. The pain may mimic angina pectoris or that of an acute myocardial infarction. It is commonly located in the chest, back, or shoulders. The dyspnea may become more severe as the patient leans forward, indicating that the teratoma is compressing the airway or the pulmonary vasculature. Less frequently, superior vena cava syndrome may develop from the mass compressing the vena cava (Fig. 5.2). Ascites, hepatomegaly, and peripheral edema have all been reported to result from compression of the vena cava by the mass [10]. Pressure on the pulmonary conus may also cause arrythmias. The tumors can perforate into the aorta, superior vena cava, or pericardium. When they perforate into the pericardium, they can cause pericarditis and tamponade [10]. They have also been

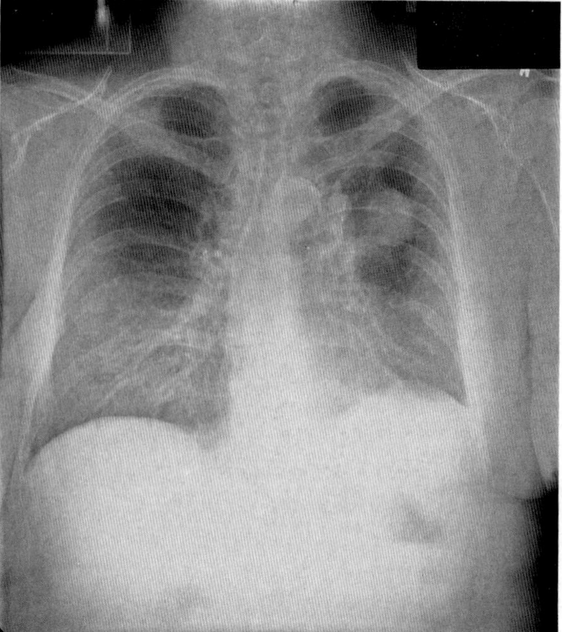

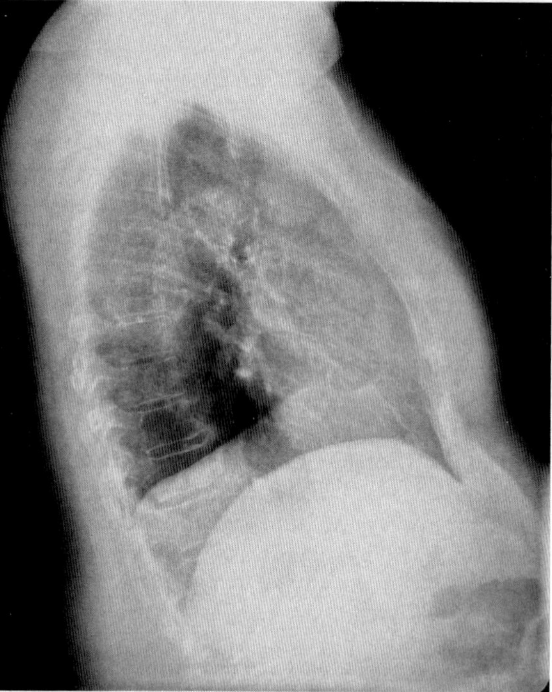

Fig. 5.1a, b. Chest roentgenograms (**a** anterior-posterior, **b** lateral) of an asymptomatic 37-year-old patient, demonstrating mediastinal teratoma

reported to perforate into the myocardium and cause a myocardial abscess.

Cough is also a relatively common symptom. This may be productive of blood, hair, or sebaceous material. When patients cough up hair (trycoptosis)

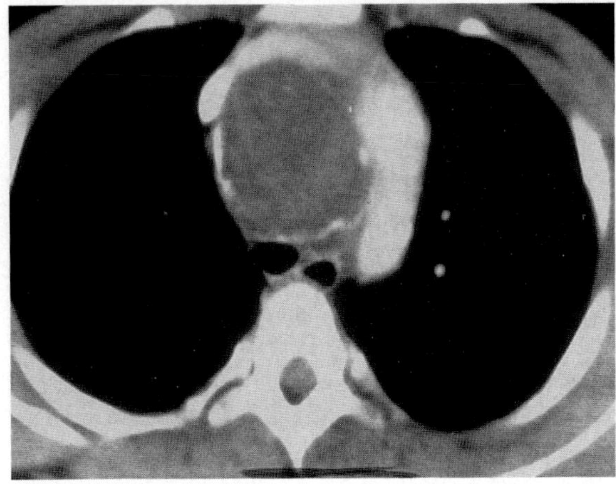

Fig. 5.2. Computed tomography of a mediastinal teratoma, demonstrating displacement and compression of the superior vena cava

or sebaceous material, this is a pathognomonic symptom. This implies that the cyst has ruptured into a bronchus, and the contents of the cyst are being expectorated. In general, the larger the mass, the more likely the patient is to have symptoms. Malignant tumors almost always are associated with symptoms, whereas less than half of the patients with benign tumors have symptoms.

The physical examination is rarely of much help in confirming the diagnosis. In LeRoux's series of 21 patients, there were five who had a visible bulge on the chest wall [8]. Two patients had loud systolic murmurs that were increased by leaning forward. These were thought to be from compression of the pulmonary artery by the tumor mass. Breath sounds may be decreased by either bronchial obstruction or the presence of a pleural effusion. Wheezing may be heard if the airway is compromised by the mass. Cyanosis or upper torso edema may also be noted. Finally, acanthosis nigricans has been associated with benign teratomas [5, 8]. Physical examination should also include careful palpation of the testes, although mediastinal teratomas are rarely associated with testicular carcinomas.

The differential diagnosis includes aortic arch aneurysm, thymoma, intrathoracic goiter, lymphoma, bronchogenic cyst, and lipoma. As in all mediastinal masses, an aortic aneurysm should be excluded. The preoperative evaluation should be directed to differentiate the different lesions in the mediastinum and to determine whether distant disease is present. After identification of the mass on chest roentgenogram, computed tomography (CT) of the chest is indicated. This yields information about the size, shape,

composition, and associations of the mass. The scan should include the upper abdomen so the liver and adrenals can be imaged. Brain and bone scans are obtained when warranted by symptoms. There is no role for blind testicular biopsy in this group of patients.

Chest roentgenogram is abnormal in more than 90% of patients with a mediastinal teratoma (Fig. 5.3). The mass is seen as a well-demarcated abnormality in the anterior mediastinum that protrudes to one side of the chest. Typically, benign germ cell tumors are rounded and lobulated. If the mass is poorly demarcated with an infiltrating border, then it is more likely to be malignant. A pleural effusion can be seen with a mediastinal teratoma [11]. Calcification is seen in 20%–40% of patients [12]. The finding of teeth on a plain chest roentgenogram is pathognomonic of a mediastinal germ cell tumor. In the Mayo series, 26% had calcification and included calcified wall, bone or teeth, and nonspecific calcification.

Computed tomography allows assessment of extent of involvement, involvement of adjacent structures, whether the mass is solid or cystic, and the pattern of calcification, if any [11] (Fig. 5.4). CT with contrast can show rim enhancement or enhancement of the tissue septa. The presence of a fat-fluid level is specific for a diagnosis of teratoma but is an unusual finding [13]. Little has been published concerning the use of magnetic resonance imaging (MRI) to diagnosis mediastinal germ cell tumors. Demonstration of an area of fat with T1-weighted images is consistent with a diagnosis of benign teratoma. Vascular compression may also be evaluated via MRI; however, the technique is too new to form many firm conclusions (Figs. 5.5, 5.6).

Laboratory evaluation is usually not helpful. Malignant germ cell tumors can have an elevated serum human chorionic gonadotropin or α-fetoprotein, but, by definition, benign tumors have negative markers. Honicky and DePapp reported a 5-year-old boy with hypoglycemia secondary to an insulin-secreting benign mediastinal teratoma [14]. However, serum blood sugar is only rarely affected by a teratoma and need not routinely be checked in the absence of symptoms.

5.5 Histology

Teratomas are true neoplasms made up of ectoderm, mesoderm, and endoderm. Although all three germ cell layers are usually present, it is possible

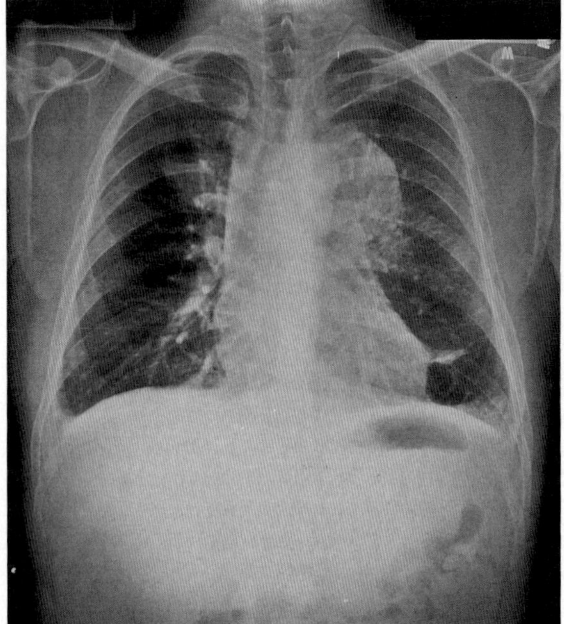

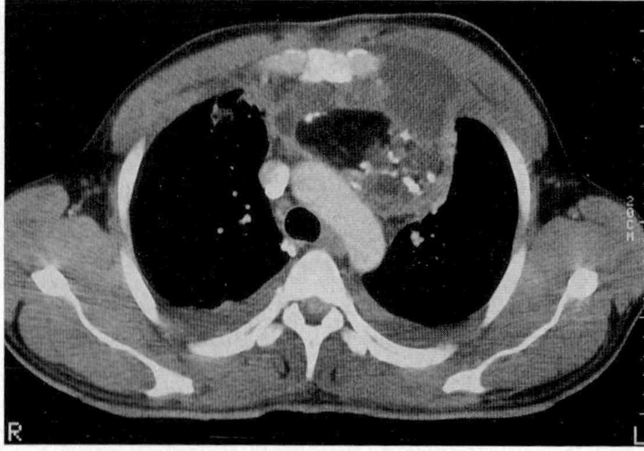

Fig. 5.4. Computed tomography demonstrating a cystic teratoma. There is also calcification seen in the left lateral aspect of the mass

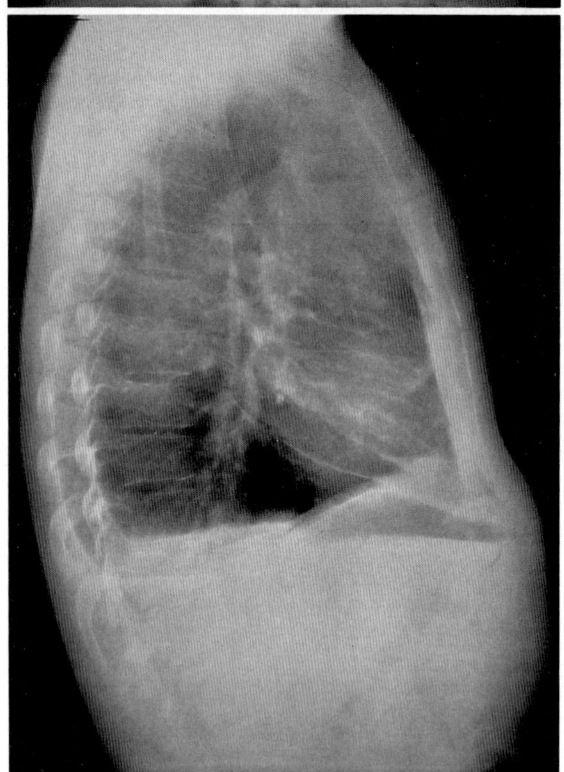

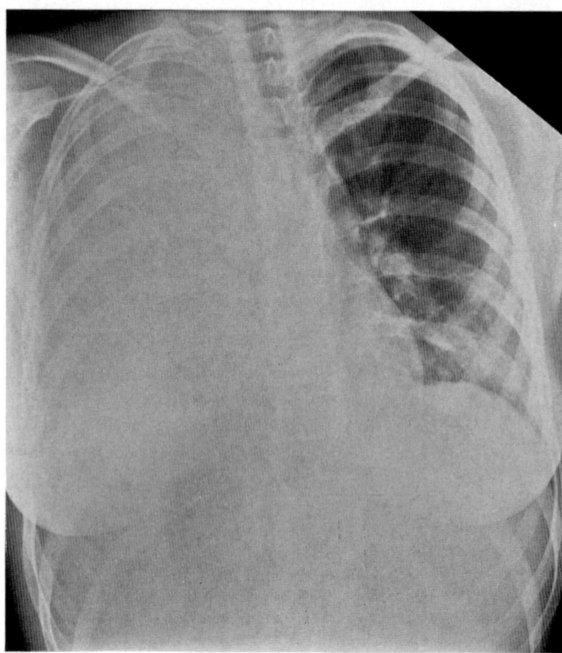

Fig. 5.5. Chest roentgenogram of a patient whose mediastinal teratoma has occluded the right main bronchus

Fig. 5.3a, b. Chest roentgenograms (a anterior-posterior, b lateral) which reveal a left anterior mediastinal mass that proved to be a teratoma at surgery

to have a monodermal or bidermal tumor; however, these are rare in the mediastinum. The capsule of a teratoma may have residual thymus tissue present. Ectoderm is represented by skin, skin appendages, and cysts lined by squamous cells. The mesoderm is represented by bone, cartilage, and muscle, and the endoderm is represented by gastrointestinal and respiratory tissue. It is possible to have malignant cells intermixed with benign tissue. These are referred to as teratocarcinoma, malignant teratoma, or mixed germ cell tumors. Sarcomas and carcinomas have rarely been described focally in a mature teratoma.

Grossly, the tumor is lobulated, spherical, and well encapsulated. The size of the tumor is variable, ranging from 2.5 to 27.0 cm [5] and from

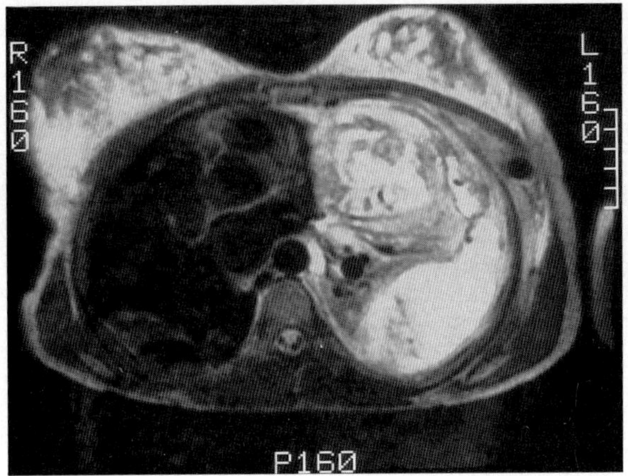

Fig. 5.6. Magnetic resonance image of the patient in Fig. 5.5, demonstrating the large anterior teratoma

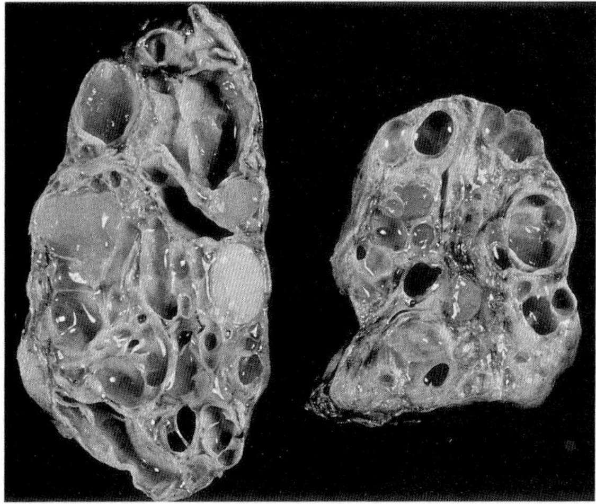

Fig. 5.7. Gross photograph of a cystic mediastinal teratoma (by permission of The Armed Forces Institute of Pathology)

25 to 1820 g. The larger the tumor, the greater the chance that a malignancy is present. The tumors are often cystic and can be filled with mucoid secretions or a yellow-white semisolid sebaceous material (Fig. 5.7). The cysts may also contain hair. Necrotic or hemorrhagic areas should be closely examined for malignancy.

5.6 Treatment and Results

The ideal treatment of a benign mediastinal germ cell tumor is complete surgical excision. All patients should undergo resection unless they are physiologically unable to tolerate it, since malig-

nant degeneration has been reported [15]. Complete resection is universally curative if the tumor is benign. The Mayo series followed 69 patients for an average of 10 years after complete resection. No patient had a recurrence; however, four patients died intraoperatively, all prior to 1945, and one died 6 months postoperatively of unknown causes. Radiation therapy has no role in the management of this tumor. In the Mayo series, seven patients received radiation therapy prior to 1951, and none of the tumors responded [5].

The surgical approach to these tumors is usually via a median sternotomy or occasionally through a posterior lateral thoracotomy [16]. Complete excision is the goal; however, there may be vital structures adherent to the tumor, making complete resection difficult. In order of decreasing frequency, the Mayo series found the tumor to be adherent to pericardium, lung, great vessels, thymus, chest wall, hilum of the lung, and diaphragm. When there is attachment to surrounding structures, it is difficult to differentiate between benign and malignant. Tumors that are adherent to surrounding structures are either malignant or are inflammatory and have eroded into the surrounding tissue. If the tumor invades lung, a wedge excision or a lobectomy may be necessary for complete resection.

The use of video-assisted thoracic surgical techniques to remove these tumors is to be condemned. Exposure is limited, and currently available equipment is unable to perform a complete resection. Until techniques and equipment improve, teratomas are best removed by open methods.

In summary, mediastinal teratomas are benign tumors which are thought to arise from pluripotent tissue that has migrated to the mediastinum during development. Patients are usually asymptomatic, and the tumor is found on a routine chest roentgenogram. The tumor is usually cystic and may contain hair or teeth. Teratomas should be completely excised, which provides a complete cure.

References

1. Rosado-de-Christenson ML, Templeton PA, Moran CA (1992) Mediastinal germ cell tumors: radiologic and pathologic correlation. Radio graphics 12: 1013–1030
2. Hainsworth JD, Greco FA (1989) Mediastinal germ cell neoplasms. In: Roth JA, Ruckdeschel JC, Weisenburger TH (eds) Thoracic oncology. Saunders, Philadelphia, pp 478–489
3. Knapp RH, Hurt RD, Payne WS, et al. (1985) Malignant germ cell tumors of the mediastinum. J Thorac Cardiovasc Surg 89: 82–89

4. Nichols CR (1992) Mediastinal germ cell tumors. Semin Thorac Cardiovasc Surg 4: 45–50
5. Lewis BD, Hurt RD, Payne S, Farrow GM, Knapp RH, Muhm JR (1983) Benign teratomas of the mediastinum. J Thorac Cardiovasc Surg 86: 727–731
6. Lack EE, Weinstein HJ, Welch KJ (1985) Mediastinal germ cell tumors in childhood. A clinical and pathological study of 21 cases. J Thorac Cardiovasc Surg 89: 826–835
7. Thomas CR, Bonomi PD (1991) Mediastinal tumors. Curr Opin Oncol 3: 335–343
8. LeRoux BT (1962) Cysts and tumors of the mediastinum. Surg Gynecol Obstet 115: 695–703
9. Gonzalez-Crussi F (1982) Atlas of tumor pathology. Extragonadal teratomas. Second series, Fascicle 18. Armed Forces Institute of Pathology, Washington DC
10. Marsten JL, Cooper AG, Ankeney JL (1966) Acute cardiac tamponade due to perforation of a benign mediastinal teratoma into the pericardial sac. Review of cardiovascular manifestations of mediastinal teratomas. J Thorac Cardiovasc Surg 51: 700–707
11. Brown LR, Muhm JR, Aughenbaugh GL, Lewis BD, Hurt RD (1987) Computed tomography of benign mature teratomas of the mediastinum. J Thorac Imaging 2: 66–71
12. Dehner LP (1990) Germ cell tumors of the mediastinum. Semin Diagn Pathol 7: 266–284
13. Weinberg B, Rose JS, Efremidis SC, Kirschner PA, Gribetz D (1980) Posterior mediastinal teratoma (cystic dermoid): diagnosis by computerized tomography. Chest 77: 694–695
14. Honicky RE, dePapp EW (1973) Mediastinal teratoma with endocrine function. Am J Dis Child 126: 650–653
15. Adebonojo SA, Nicola ML (1976) Teratoid tumors of the mediastinum. Am Surg 43: 361–365
16. Ferguson MK, Lee E, Skinner DB, Little AG (1987) Selective operative approach for diagnosis and treatment of anterior mediastinal masses. Ann Thorac Surg 44: 583–586

6 Nonseminomatous Germ Cell Tumors of the Mediastinum

CAMERON D. WRIGHT, JOHN C. WAIN, and DOUGLAS J. MATHISEN

CONTENTS

6.1 Introduction

Nonseminomatous germ cell tumors of the mediastinum represent a rare subset of both mediastinal tumors and germ cell cancer. Before cisplatin-based chemotherapy, the outlook for these patients was grim. Recent reports utilizing cisplatin-based chemotherapy with adjuvant surgery when necessary have demonstrated a considerable improvement in outcome.

6.2 Etiology

Nonseminomatous germ cell tumors of the mediastinum are thought to arise as a consequence of an error of migration of germ cells along the urogenital ridge during embryogenesis [1]. An alternative hypothesis is that these neoplasms arise from a rest of totipotential cells that occur during normal embryogenesis [2]. An older hypothesis since discarded suggested that these tumors were metastatic deposits from unrecognized testicular tumors [3].

6.3 Incidence

Nonseminomatous germ cell tumors of the mediastinum are uncommon and represent only 1%–3% of all tumors of the mediastinum [4, 5]. Mediastinal germ cell tumors account for only 1%–3% of all germinal tumors as well [6]. However, mediastinal germ cell tumors are the most common extragonadal site among germ cell tumors [7]. More than 90% of nonseminomatous germ cell tumors occur in men [8]. There is a wide variation in age at presentation, with children being affected as well as adults in their sixth decade of life. The average age of presentation is 30 [8].

6.4 Pathology

Nonseminomatous germ cell tumors of the mediastinum appear similar histologically to testicular germ cell tumors. Teratocarcinoma (teratoma with embryonal cell carcinoma) is the most common histologic type [9]. Other histologic types seen include pure embryonal cell carcinoma, pure endodermal sinus tumor (yolk sac tumor), choriocarcinoma, and mixed nonseminomatous histologies.

6.5 Clinical Characteristics

Characteristically the symptoms are of short duration as these tumors grow rapidly. Symptoms are commonly produced by the presence of a large mass in the anterior mediastinum and include chest pain, cough, and shortness of breath. Constitutional symptoms of fever and weight loss are also common. Physical examination is usually normal, but

CAMERON D. WRIGHT, M.D., Assistant Professor of Surgery, Harvard Medical School; Assistant Surgeon, General Thoracic Surgical Services, Warren 1212, Massachusetts General Hospital, Boston, MA 02114, USA
JOHN C. WAIN, M.D., Assistant Professor of Surgery, Harvard Medical School; Director, Lung Transplant Program, General Thoracic Surgical Services, Massachusetts General Hospital, Boston, MA 02114, USA
DOUGLAS J. MATHISEN, M.D., Associate Professor of Surgery, Harvard Medical School; Associate Visiting Surgeon, General Thoracic Surgical Services, Massachusetts General Hospital, Boston, MA 02114, USA

occasionally supraclavicular adenopathy is palpable; stigmata of the superior vena cava syndrome are occasionally seen and gynecomastia is rarely present.

Chest radiographs typically show a large anterior superior mediastinal mass (Fig. 6.1). The chest radiograph is almost always abnormal in these patients. Computed tomography (CT) usually shows a large inhomogeneous mass with multiple areas of necrosis and hemorrhage (Fig. 6.2). Compression of mediastinal structures is commonly seen, as is invasion of adjacent structures and envelopment of blood vessels.

Measurement of the serum tumor markers β-human chorionic gonadotropin (HCG) and α-fetoprotein (AFP) is indispensable in the management of nonseminomatous germ cell tumors. These markers should be measured when evaluating an anterior mediastinal mass, especially in a young person. Approximately 90% of patients with nonseminomatous mediastinal germ cell tumors will have elevation of one or both of these markers [8]. About 80% have elevated AFP levels and 30% have elevated HCG levels. Primary mediastinal seminomas may occasionally be associated with mild elevation of β-HCG levels (< 100). If there is a significant elevation in AFP levels then nonseminomatous elements are present within the tumor

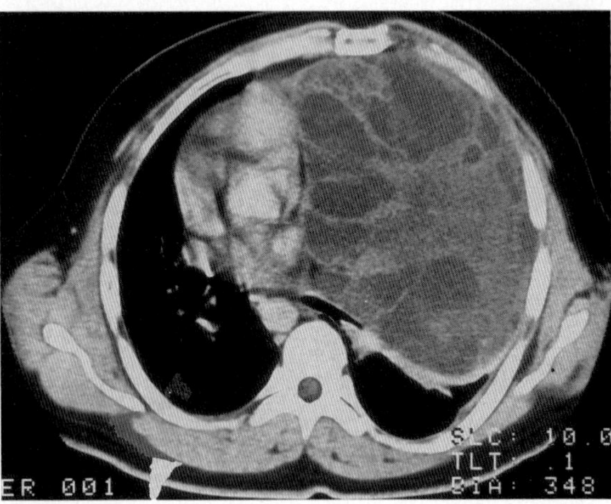

Fig. 6.2. CT scan of same patient as in Fig. 6.1 reveals a large inhomogeneous tumor filling the left hemithorax, compressing lung and shifting the mediastinum to the right

and it should be reclassified as a nonseminomatous tumor. In addition, lactate dehydrogenase (LDH) is elevated in approximately 90% of these patients and serial determinations are useful in following the activity of the tumor.

6.6 Pretreatment Evaluation

Evaluation should include a history, especially searching for symptoms compatible with occult metastatic disease. Physical examination should also include a careful testis examination to make sure one is not dealing with an unrecognized testicular primary. Routine ultrasound examination or biopsy of the testes is not indicated. Computed tomography of the chest and abdomen should be performed and AFP, HCG, and LDH levels should be measured. Bone or brain scans are not performed unless symptoms warrant them. Pulmonary function tests with measurement of the diffusing capacity are indicated if bleomycin therapy is anticipated.

Surgical confirmation of the diagnosis is preferred, but not absolutely mandatory. In institutions with an experienced cytopathologist a fine-needle aspiration (FNA) is the preferred approach. A limited anterior mediastinotomy (Chamberlain procedure) is the preferred route of surgical biopsy if FNA is not feasible. Thoracotomy should be avoided as it delays institution of required chemotherapy. Biopsy is useful to provide the precise histology of the tumor (which may have prognostic implications) and can also document non-germ cell

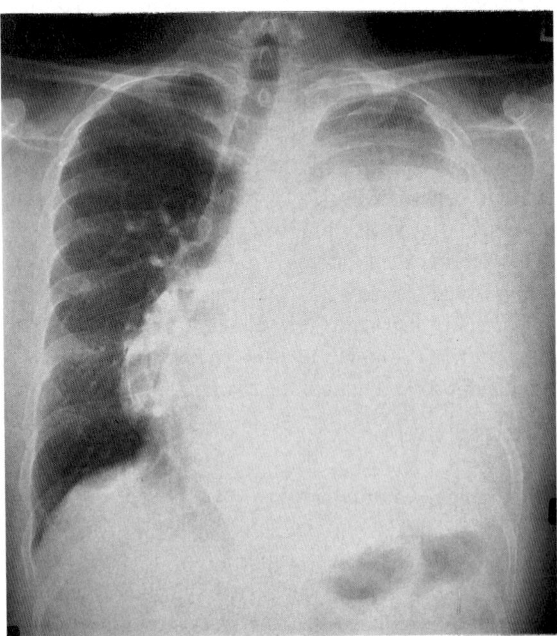

Fig. 6.1. Chest radiograph of a young man with yolk sac carcinoma demonstrating a massive mediastinal tumor presenting in the left hemithorax with pleural effusion and mediastinal shift

elements which are occasionally seen with these tumors. Chemotherapy can be instituted without delay based solely on the clinical presentation of a mediastinal tumor with elevation of serum tumor markers in patients who present with far-advanced disease.

6.7 Treatment

Local treatment modalities have not proven effective in treatment of nonseminomatous mediastinal germ cell tumors. The results of primary radiation therapy are poor, with a high incidence of both local failure and systemic recurrence [10]. Surgical therapy alone also is of little benefit and rarely provides long-term survivers [11]. Furthermore, results with single-agent or non-cisplatin-based chemotherapy are likewise poor [11].

Cisplatin-based chemotherapy has dramatically improved the survival of patients with testicular germ cell cancers and now provides cure rates in excess of 70% in these patients [12]. Survival rates are related to the volume of disease at presentation [13]. Patients with nonseminomatous mediastinal germ cell tumors are similar to patients with testicular germ cell cancer in the poor prognosis category as they have a large bulk of disease at presentation. Not surprisingly, the survival of patients with mediastinal nonseminomatous germ cell cancers is quite similar to that of their counterparts with advanced testicular germ cell cancer [9].

Cisplatin-based chemotherapy should be administered for 3–4 cycles over a 3- to 4-month span. Severe treatment toxicity is unusual. The patient should be restaged with repeat computed tomography and marker studies performed at the end of treatment. A complete response (normal serum tumor markers and normal radiographs) is the goal of treatment. Figure 6.3 summarizes the management of these patients following induction chemotherapy. If the serum tumor markers and the radiographs normalize, observation only is warranted. There is an approximate 20% relapse rate from a complete response and most relapses occur within the first 2 years [8, 9]. Careful follow-up is mandatory with monthly office visits, radiographs, and serum tumor marker evaluations performed for the first year and then every 2 months for the second year.

Patients with persistent elevation of their serum tumor markers have residual active carcinoma and should receive salvage chemotherapy. Nonetheless, salvage chemotherapy rarely yields long-term survival [8]. Treatment of these patients with high-dose chemotherapy and autologous bone marrow rescue has likewise been disappointing [14].

Patients with normalization of markers after chemotherapy and persistent abnormalities on radiographs should undergo surgical resections to classify further their response to treatment. The

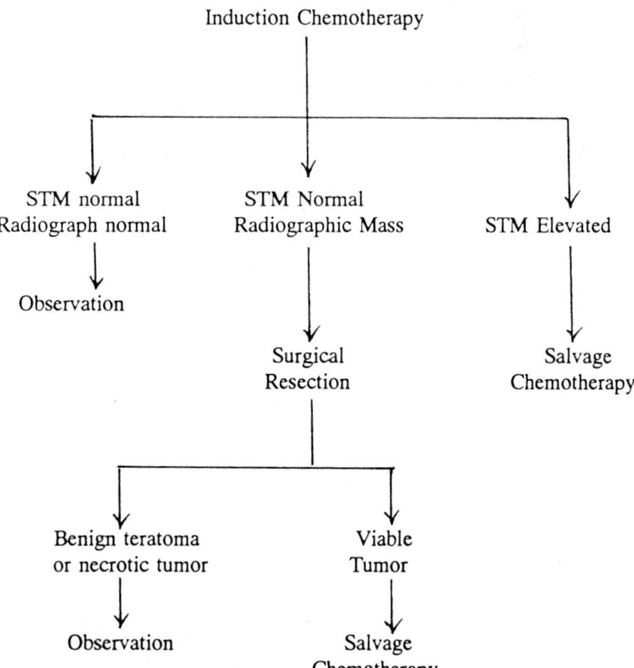

Fig. 6.3. Management of nonseminomatous germ cell tumors of the mediastinum after induction chemotherapy. *STM*, serum tumor markers

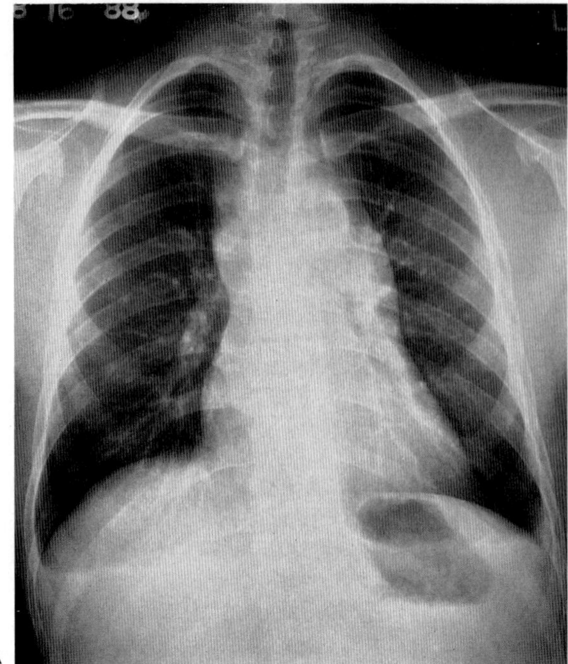

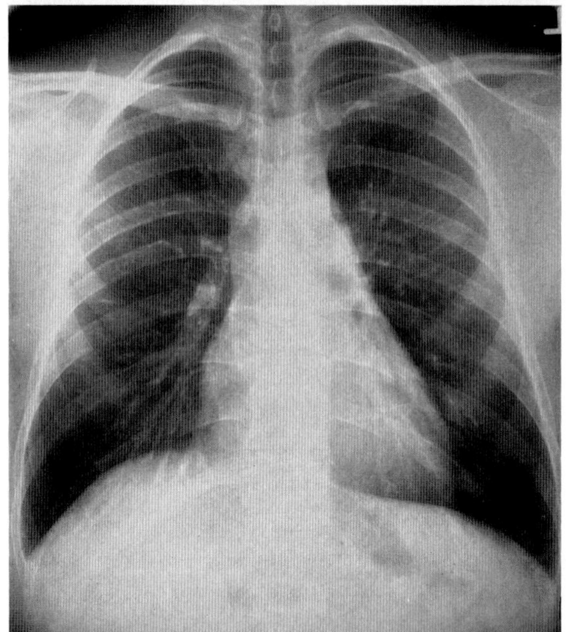

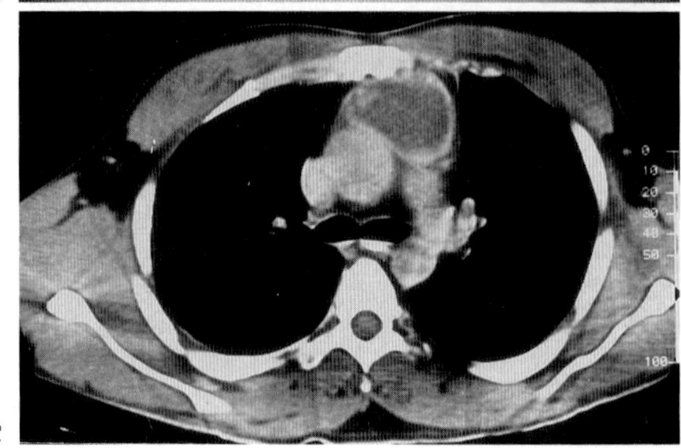

majority of patients treated with cisplatin chemotherapy are in this category and need adjunctive surgery to obtain a complete response [8]. More than 50% of these patients will have benign teratoma in the resected specimen [8, 9]. The response to induction chemotherapy in a typical patient who required subsequent resection to obtain a complete response is illustrated in Fig. 6.4. Residual mass should be removed to exclude the possibility of residual marker-negative germ cell cancer or malignant non-germ cell elements and to prevent future problems with teratoma. Teratoma may exhibit slow local growth which can compress or eventually invade vital structures and has been reported to undergo malignant degeneration [15]. Those patients who are noted to have a large amount of teratoma on their preoperative biopsy specimens have a greater likelihood of needing surgery to remove persistent teratoma after chemotherapy. Patients with viable tumor in the resected specimen should receive salvage chemotherapy. Patients with non-germ cell tumor in the resected specimen have a poor prognosis and the treatment of these patients is uncertain and individualized. Patients who have no viable germ cell cancer in the resected specimen should be observed as described previously.

Median sternotomy is the incision of choice for tumors present primarily in the midline. Often the tumors will present as predominantly hemithorax masses and in such cases the standard posterolateral thoracotomy or transsternal anterior thoracotomy is the incision of choice. Partial pericardiectomy is usually required as these tumors are usually intimately adherent to the anterior surface of the pericardium. Phrenic nerve involvement is not uncommon and if possible the phrenic nerve should be preserved if the attachment is peripheral and thought to be due to fibrosis. This can be confirmed with frozen section analysis. If there is significant involvement of the phrenic nerve, however, it should be sacrificed as benign teratoma left in this area can cause significant problems years later. Major vascular resections should be avoided as these tumors are

Fig. 6.4A–C. Embryonal cell carcinoma in a young man. A Chest radiograph prior to treatment demonstrates a mediastinal mass. B Chest radiograph of the same patient after three cycles of cisplatin-based chemotherapy. Only partial resolution of the mediastinal mass has occurred although the serum tumor markers have returned to normal. C CT scan after four cycles of cisplatin-based chemotherapy reveals a small residual encapsulated anterior mediastinal tumor. Resection revealed necrotic tumor and benign teratoma only

Table 6.1. Nonseminomatous mediastinal germ cell tumors: results with cisplatin-based chemotherapy

Authors	Year	Patients	No. of surgical resections	Complete response	Survival
KAY et al.	1987	10	7	60%	40% (4 yrs)
WRIGHT et al.	1990	28	20	79%	57% (5 yrs)
LEMARIE et al.	1992	45	22	64%	53% (2 yrs)

usually surrounded by a pseudocapsule which allows them to be removed from major vessels without a great deal of difficulty. Not uncommonly, there will be a firm attachment to an upper lobe of the lung and either wedge resection or upper lobectomy is necessary. Postoperative complications are rare in the usual young patient.

6.8 Prognosis

Long-term survival within intensive cisplatin regimens currently approaches 50% at 5 years. This is a dramatic improvement as compared to previous treatment modalities. Because of the limited numbers of patients it is difficult to assign a prognostic value to various histologic subtypes of nonseminomatous mediastinal germ cell cancers. Historically, yolk sac tumors and choriocarcinomas have been associated with a poorer prognosis than other subtypes [9]. Multiple centers now report similar long-term survival rates despite minor differences in chemotherapy regimens [8, 16, 17] (Table 6.1). Further improvements in therapy are needed as survival of this group of patients is still distinctly inferior to that of the typical patient with testicular germ cell cancer.

References

1. Willis RA (1962) Borderland of embryology and pathology, 2nd edn. Butterworth, Washington DC, pp 442
2. Schlumberger HG (1946) Teratoma of anterior mediastinum in group of military age: study of 16 cases and review of theories of genesis. Arch Pathol 41: 398–444
3. Luna MA, Valenznela-Tamariz J (1976) Germ cell tumors of the mediastinum. Post-mortem findings. Am J Clin Pathol 65: 450–454
4. Davis RD, Oldham HN, Sabistan DC (1987) Primary cysts and neoplasms of the mediastinum: recent changes in clinical presentation, methods of diagnosis, management, and results. Ann Thorac Surg 44: 229–237
5. Wychulis AR, Payne WS, Clagett OT, Woolner LB (1971) Surgical treatment of mediastinal tumor: a 40 year experience. J Thorac Cardiovasc Surg 62: 379–391
6. Collins DH, Pugh RCB (1964) Classification and frequency of testicular tumors. Br J Urol 361 (suppl): 1–11
7. Kuhn MW, Weissbach L (1985) Localization, incidence, diagnosis and treatment of extratesticular germ cell tumors. Urol Int 40: 166–172
8. Wright CD, Kesler KA, Nichols CR, Mahomed Y, et al. (1990) Primary mediastinal nonseminomatous germ cell tumors. Results of a multimodality approach. J Thorac Cardiovasc Surg 99: 210–217
9. Hainsworth JD, Greco FA (1991) General features of malignant germ cell tumors and primary seminomas of the mediastinum. In: Shields TW (ed) Mediastinal surgery, 1st edn. Lea and Febiger, Philadelphia, pp 211–218
10. Kersh CR, Eisert DR, Constable WC, Hahn SS, et al. (1987) Primary malignant mediastinal germ cell tumors and the contribution of radiotherapy: a southeastern multi-institutional study. Am J Clin Oncol 10: 302–306
11. Economou JS, Trump DL, Holmes EC, Eggleston JE (1982) Management of primary germ cell tumors of the mediastinum. J Thorac Cardiovasc Surg 83: 643–649
12. Hainsworth JD, Greco FA (1983) Testicular germ cell neoplasms. Am J Med 75: 817–832
13. Birch R, Williams S, Cone A, et al. (1986) Prognostic factors for favorable outcome in disseminated germ cell tumors. J Clin Oncol 4: 400–407
14. Broun ER, Nichols CR, Kneebone P, Williams SA (1992) Long-term outcome of patients with relapsed and refractory germ cell tumors treated with high-dose chemotherapy and autologous bone marrow rescue. Ann Intern Med 117: 124–128
15. Loehrer PJ, Hui S, Clark SA, et al. (1986) Teratoma following cisplatin-based combination chemotherapy for nonseminomatous germ cell tumor: a clinicopathological correlation. J Urol 135: 1183–1189
16. Kay PH, Wells FC, Goldstraw P (1987) A multidisciplinary approach to primary nonseminomatous germ cell tumors of the mediastinum. Ann Thorac Surg 44: 578–582
17. Lemarie E, Assouline PS, Diot P, Regnard JF, et al. (1992) Primary mediastinal germ cell tumors. Results of a French retrospective study. Chest 102: 1477–1483

7 Primary Mediastinal Seminoma

RICHARD F. HEITMILLER and WILLIAM J. MARASCO

CONTENTS

7.1 Etiology

The histologic appearance of primary mediastinal and testicular seminomas is identical; therefore it is always important to rule out metastatic testicular disease in patients with suspected primary mediastinal seminoma. The histogenic origin of extragonadal germ cell tumors has been a matter of controversy. In 1946 SCHLUMBERGER proposed that these tumors were of thymic origin and were the result of disordered somatic cell development [1]. This theory failed to explain the presence of germinomatous elements in mixed tumors which could not have arisen from somatic tissue [2]. Others have argued that mediastinal seminoma represents metastatic disease, and that the primary testicular tumor is either occult or has undergone spontaneous regression. Clinical and postmortem studies do not support the theory of metastatic mediastinal disease from an occult testicular primary. In addition the theory does not explain the finding of mediastinal seminoma in women. In 1951, FRIEDMAN proposed a theory supporting the existence of primary extragonadal germ cell tumors which has become generally accepted [3]. The theory states that displaced primordial germ cells, which are located along the midline, are the origin for all extragonadal germ cell tumors. In this theory, the different morphologic patterns of germ cell tumors resulted from different stages of tumor differentiation.

7.2 Demographics

Primary mediastinal seminoma, like germ cell tumors as a whole, is almost exclusively a disease of males. Reports of mediastinal seminomas in women are infrequent enough to prompt case reports [4]. These tumors occur most commonly in patients in their third decade, followed by patients in their second and fourth decades. Both malignant germ cell tumors in general, and primary mediastinal seminoma in particular, occur over a broad age range [5]. The age distribution for women with mediastinal seminoma appears to be the same as with males. Primary mediastinal seminoma is more common in whites than blacks. AYGUN et al. [6], in their collective review, noted only one black patient out of 26 patients in which race was mentioned. The incidence of mediastinal germ cell tumors is increased in patients with Klinefelter's syndrome, with non-seminomatous tumors predominating [7].

7.3 Incidence

Germ cell tumors account for 10%–15% of all mediastinal cysts and tumors in adults [8]. In their series, MULLEN and RICHARDSON [9] reported that germ cell tumors accounted for 24% of mediastinal tumors in children. If only malignant mediastinal tumors are considered, the incidence of germ cell tumors is as high as 28.9% [10].

RICHARD F. HEITMILLER, M.D., Assistant Professor of Surgery, Division of General Thoracic Surgery, Osler 624, Johns Hopkins Hospital, 600 N. Wolfe St., Baltimore, MD 21205, USA

WILLIAM J. MARASCO, M.D., Russell H. Morgan Department of Radiology and Radiological Science, Johns Hopkins Medical Institution, 600 N. Wolfe St., Baltimore, MD 21205, USA

Mediastinal germ cell tumors include seminoma, teratoma, embryonal cell, choriocarcinoma, and yolk sac (endodermal sinus) tumors. Germ cell tumors may comprise a single cell type ("pure") or contain a mixture of cell types. Pure mediastinal seminomas are more common than mixed seminomas [2], and represent 39%–48% of mediastinal germ cell tumors [2, 11]. By extrapolating the above figures, it can be estimated that the incidence of mediastinal seminoma in adults may be as high as 5%–7%, and that the majority of these tumors will be pure seminomas.

7.4 Diagnosis

7.4.1 Clinical Features

Primary mediastinal tumors are usually bulky, and have a tendency to invade or encircle adjacent mediastinal structures. However, the symptoms caused by these bulky tumors are usually nonspecific [12–14]. Symptoms are often unimpressive when contrasted with the extent of the tumor [15]. The most common symptom is chest pain, followed by respiratory symptoms such as dyspnea and cough. Although there are several reports of hemoptysis with nonseminomatous germ cell tumors [2, 16, 17], it is rare in patients with primary mediastinal seminoma [18]. Dysphagia and hoarseness are un-

common. Local invasion with superior vena caval obstruction has been reported [2]. Mediastinal seminoma may metastasize to bone, lung, liver, spleen, tonsil, thyroid, skin, spinal cord, and brain [19], resulting in a spectrum of symptoms depending on the specific metastatic site.

7.4.2 Laboratory Tests and Histology

Most routine blood and urine studies are of little value. α–Fetoprotein (AFP), human chorionic gonadotropin, carcinoembryonic antigen, and serum lactic dehydrogenase may be elevated in patients with mediastinal seminomas [2]. However, histologic diagnosis is necessary in all patients despite positive tumor markers. The chief value of tumor markers is in serial follow-up determinations to define response and to detect occult recurrence [14]. On histologic examination, seminomas consist of uniform seminoma cells (Fig. 7.1) with prominent nucleoli, clear cytoplasm, and distinct cell membranes. There is also associated fibrous tissue usually containing infiltrating lymphocytes. On occasion, an inflammatory response consisting of infiltrating lymphocytes and macrophages is seen within the tumor, perhaps reflecting an immune response to the tumor. It has been suggested that this inflammatory reaction is associated with a better prognosis [20].

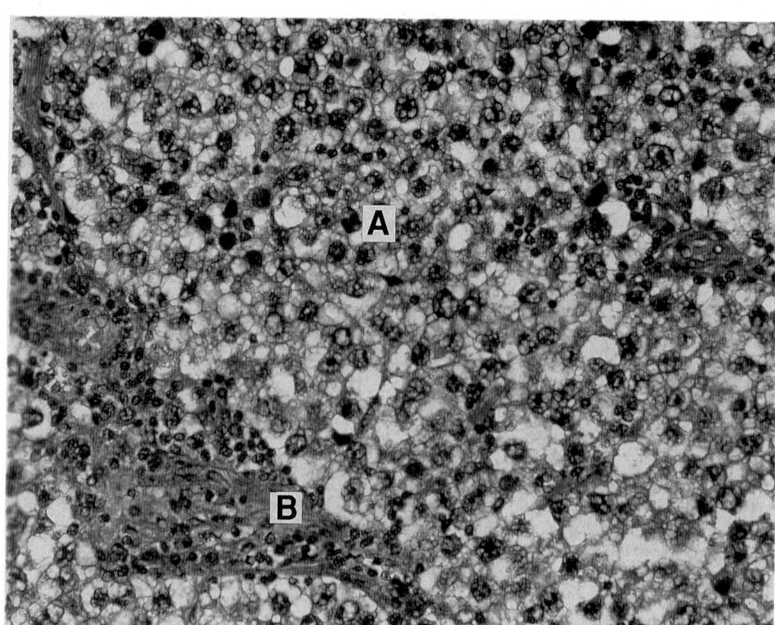

Fig. 7.1. Photomicrograph of seminoma demonstrating uniform population of seminoma cells (*A*) with characteristic prominent nucleoli, clear cytoplasm, and distinct cell membranes. The typical fibrous tissue with infiltrating lymphocytes (*B*) is also demonstrated. ×250

7.4.3 Radiology

Due to the size of the mediastinal tumors, the diagnosis of a mediastinal mass is usually made on routine chest roentgenograms (Fig. 7.2). In addition to plain chest films, we feel that chest computered tomography (CT) (Fig. 7.3) should be performed to define the tumor size, determine the presence and extent of mediastinal invasion, and detect lymphadenopathy and pulmonary metastasis. Chest CT is also useful to accurately plan radiation therapy ports [21], and serial scans may be used to monitor the response to therapy. Abdominal CT is recommended to determine the extent of disease below the diaphragm. Extensive retroperitoneal lymphadenopathy may suggest a testicular primary. Ultrasound examination of the testis should be performed, and, if a suspicious lesion is seen, either testicular biopsy or orchiectomy considered [22]. Other investigations such as a radionuclide bone scan or CT of the head may be performed if symptoms suggest metastatic disease.

7.5 Staging and Prognostic Factors

The staging systems which are now used for testicular seminomas are modifications of the Boden and Gibb staging which was first proposed in 1951

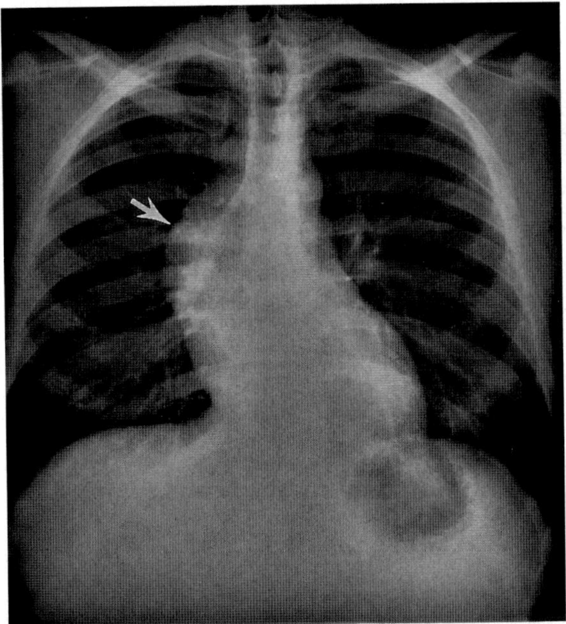

Fig. 7.2. Chest film revealing a large right mediastinal mass (*arrow*) in the suprahilar region

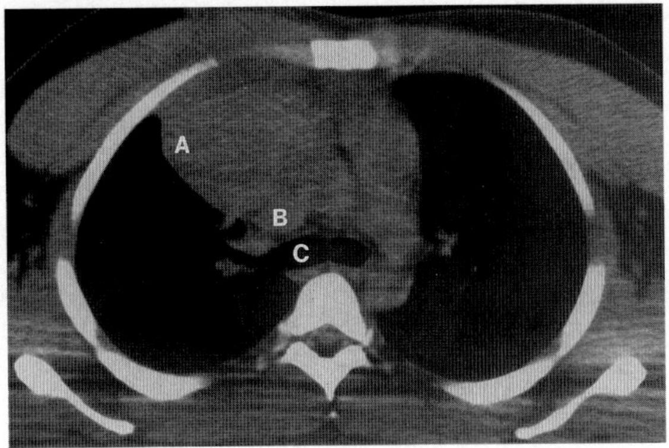

Fig. 7.3. Unenhanced thoracic CT scan at the level of the carina demonstrating a large anterior mediastinal mass (*A*) which compromises the superior vena cava (*B*) and airway (*C*)

[23]. There is no widely acceptable staging system for patients with primary extragonadal seminoma. Whereas some advocate using the testicular seminoma staging systems for all patients with seminoma, CEFARO et al. [24] proposed a separate staging classification for these patients. In their system, which is outlined in Table 7.1, stage I is localized disease, stage II is bulky mediastinal disease which compresses but does not invade mediastinal structures, stage III disease is locally invasive, and stage IV represents metastatic disease. We agree that a separate staging scheme for patients with primary mediastinal seminoma is warranted, and that the classification proposed by CEFARO et al. [24], which is based on parameters important in treatment and prognosis, should be adopted.

Reported poor prognostic factors, many of which are reflected in the proposed staging system listed above, include age greater than 35 years, bulky mediastinal disease which is not amenable to complete resection, superior vena caval obstruction, lymphadenopathy, hilar disease, and elevated AFP levels [2, 25].

7.6 Therapy

Therapy for mediastinal seminoma has not been standardized because of the relative rarity of the disease, the ability of the disease to present as localized (with or without invasion) or metastatic disease, the paucity of prospective randomized clinical trials, and the lack of a unified staging system. As experience in the management of these tumors grows, it becomes increasingly clear that the

Table 7.1. Summary of staging system for primary mediastinal seminoma as proposed by CEFARO et al. [24]

Stage I	Localized
Stage II	Bulky, noninvasive
Stage III	Locally invasive
Stage IV	Metastatic

treatment principles and results parallel those of primary testicular seminoma. The individual treatment options and results are discussed separately below.

7.6.1 Surgery

Surgical options include complete resection, tumor debulking, and biopsy. The majority of patients with mediastinal seminoma present with symptoms reflecting a locally invasive tumor which is not amenable to complete surgical resection. Both KNAPP et al. [2] and AYGUN et al. [6] reported successful resection in only 37.5% of patients with mediastinal seminoma. In addition, even in patients with noninvasive localized disease, surgery alone has proven inadequate. Although complete surgical resection is advocated whenever possible, adjuvant therapy, usually radiation therapy, is considered standard. The preferred surgical approach utilizes a median sternotomy incision.

KIFFER and SAUDEMAN [26] reported that, in their experience, surgical debulking of mediastinal seminomas followed by postoperative radiation therapy yielded the best results. Their series was small (four patients), and unusual in that 75% of patients could be resected with "macroscopic clearance" of tumor. KERSH et al. [11], in a larger series of 13 patients all of whom received mediastinal irradiation, reported survival by extent of preradiation surgical resection, and noted 100% survival in those patients in whom complete resection had been performed. Patients undergoing open biopsy or subtotal resections had survivals which were not significantly different, but poorer than the complete resection group. In most reports, even though surgical resection or debulking has often been performed in patients treated with radiation therapy or chemotherapy, it is not clear that surgery has enhanced local control or survival by comparison with nonoperative management.

Surgery is used mostly to biopsy the mediastinal tumor to establish the diagnosis. A biopsy can be performed using a median sternotomy or a paratracheal or thoracoscopic approach.

7.6.2 Radiation Therapy

Like testicular seminoma, primary mediastinal seminoma is sensitive to radiation therapy. There are numerous studies which demonstrate the effectiveness of radiation therapy in the management of patients with disease localized to the mediastinum, with or without local invasion, either as the sole therapy or following surgical resection [2, 6, 11, 25, 26]. The recommended radiation dose varies from 30 to 45 Gy. Although some recommend higher doses, the data do not suggest that this is necessary. KERSH et al. [11] generated a dose-response curve based on a total radiation dose ranging from 30 to 50 Gy. They noted only one local control failure, in a patient receiving 45 Gy, and concluded that for primary mediastinal seminoma, doses higher than 30 Gy may not be required.

In order for radiation therapy to be effective, an adequate treatment field must be used which includes the entire mediastinum and supraclavicular lymph nodes. UEMATSU et al. [27] demonstrated no local recurrence in patients receiving whole mediastinal and supraclavicular radiation, whereas two-thirds of those patients receiving limited field radiation relapsed locally. In addition, in their series, locally recurrent disease proved to be relatively resistant to salvage therapy.

Overall, radiation therapy is reported to achieve local tumor control in 89%–97% of patients with mediastinal seminoma [6, 27]. In addition to its effectiveness in treating primary mediastinal disease, radiation therapy is also effective in managing symptomatic metastasis. LEE and JACKSON [28] reported one long-term survivor after radiotherapy to treat a symptomatic vertebral metastasis 1 year after mediastinal irradiation for primary mediastinal seminoma.

The reported 5-year survival following radiation therapy ranges from 50% to as high as 100% [11] in patients with localized, noninvasive disease. Most commonly, 5-year survival rates of 50%–75% [25] are reported using radiation therapy as the primary therapy.

7.6.3 Chemotherapy

Based on the favorable results obtained using cisplatin-based regimens in treating patients with advanced stage testicular carcinoma [29], many investigators have used similar regimens to treat patients with primary mediastinal seminoma.

Chemotherapeutic agents commonly employed include cisplatin, bleomycin, vinblastine, etoposide, cyclophosphamide, and doxorubicin. The most common combination regimen used is cisplatin, bleomycin, and etoposide or vinblastine. The reported complete response rates vary from 71% [30] to as high as 100% [15]. MOTZER et al. [29], using a cisplatin-based regimen, emphasized that their complete response rate of 88% was identical to that seen when treating patients with advanced stage testicular seminoma.

In the only prospective randomized trial comparing radiation therapy with chemotherapy to treat patients with extragonadal seminoma, JAIN et al. [15] demonstrated improved survival using initial chemotherapy employing high-dose cisplatin chemotherapy. In their series, 20 of 21 patients had extensive local disease, and 14 of 21 (evenly distributed between the two treatment arms) had metastasis at the time of treatment. On the basis of this single study it is unreasonable to generalize that chemotherapy is more effective primary therapy for all patients with mediastinal seminoma; however, the results do suggest that patients with locally advanced mediastinal or metastatic disease appear to benefit from initial high-dose chemotherapy.

A partial response following chemotherapy may be converted to a complete response using adjuvant radiotherapy [25]; however, especially in patients receiving bleomycin, the risk of combined treatment complications, including fatal pulmonary fibrosis, is increased.

It is not clear that a residual mass following chemotherapy mandates additional therapy. SHULTZ et al. [31] reported their experience with 21 patients with residual radiographic masses after combination cisplatin chemotherapy for advanced stage seminoma. With no additional therapy, only one patient died of recurrent disease, and two patients relapsed but were alive after 21 and 24 months respectively. The size of the residual mass did not correlate with outcome. The authors concluded that close observation with serial CT scans was a viable alternative to adjuvant therapy (or surgical biopsy) in patients with residual radiographic masses after chemotherapy. In their series, additional therapy was reserved for patients who demonstrated radiographic progression of disease.

When chemotherapy is used as the primary treatment, 5-year survival rates of 67%–85% are reported [29, 30, 32]. The posttreatment survival rates for mediastinal seminoma are the same as for patients with advanced stage testicular seminoma.

Table 7.2. Recommended treatment for patients with primary mediastinal seminoma by stage

Stage	Treatment
I	Resection, XRT
II	XRT or chemotherapy
III	XRT or chemotherapy
IV	Chemotherapy

XRT, radiation therapy

The specific recommendations for treatment are still in evolution; however, the data support the following guidelines, which are summarized in Table 7.2. The majority of patients will not present with disease amenable to complete resection. However, surgical resection of localized, noninvasive mediastinal seminomas (stage 1) should be performed whenever possible, followed by adjuvant radiation therapy. Radiation therapy has proven itself useful in the management of localized mediastinal disease (stage I, II, or III) with or without pretherapy surgical resection. In patients with extensive metastatic disease (stage IV), radiation therapy should only be used to palliate symptomatic metastasis. Whether mediastinal radiation therapy or systemic chemotherapy is the optimal therapy in patients with bulky mediastinal disease (stage II) is unproven. Chemotherapy is useful in the management of patients with extensive local disease (both stage II and stage III) or metastatic tumors (stage IV). Adjuvant radiation therapy may salvage patients who achieve a partial response from the initial chemotherapy; however, the toxicity of combined chemotherapy and radiation therapy is increased. A residual mass after chemotherapy does not mandate adjuvant therapy. Patients may be followed, reserving additional therapy for cases where progression of disease is documented radiographically. Regardless of the treatment used, long-term follow-up is required as late recurrence is possible [33].

References

1. Schlumberger HG (1946) Teratoma of anterior mediastinum in group of military age: study of sixteen cases and review of theories of genesis. Arch Pathol 41: 398–444
2. Knapp RH, Hunt RD, Payne WS, et al. (1985) Malignant germ cell tumors of the mediastinum. J Thorac Cardiovasc Surg 89: 82–89
3. Friedman NB (1951) The comparative morphogenesis of extragenital and gonadal teratoid tumors. Cancer 4: 265–276

4. Brown K, Collins JD, Betra P, Streckel RJ, Kagan AR (1989) Mediastinal germ cell tumor in a young woman. Med Pediatr Oncol 17: 164–167
5. Aggerwal P, Sharma SK, Sharma ML, Sawhney S, Aserwel J (1988) Mediastinal seminoma. A case report and review of the literature. Urol Int 43: 344–346
6. Aygun C, Slawson RG, Bajaj K, Salazar OM (1984) Primary mediastinal seminoma. Urology 23: 109–117
7. Hasle H, Jacobsen BB, Asschenfeldt P, Andersen K (1992) Mediastinal germ cell tumour associated with Klinefelter syndrome. A report of case and review of literature. Eur J Ped 151: 735–739
8. Davis RD Jr, Oldham HN Jr, Sabistaon DC Jr (1987) Primary cysts and neoplasma of the mediastinum: recent changes in clinical presentation, methods of diagnosis, management and results. Ann Thorac Surg 44: 229–237
9. Mullen B, Richardson JD (1986) Primary anterior mediastinal tumors in children and adults. Ann Thorac Surg 42: 338–345
10. Adkins RB Jr, Maples MD, Hainsworth JD (1984) Primary malignant mediastinal tumors. Ann Thorac Surg 38: 648–659
11. Kersh CR, Eisert DR, Constable WC, Hahn SS, Jenrette JM, Fitzgerald RH, Graydon J (1987) Primary malignant mediastinal germ cell tumors and the contribution of radiotherapy: a southeastern multi-institutional study. Am J Clin Oncol 10: 302–306
12. Cox JD (1975) Primary malignant germinal tumors of the mediastinum – a study of 24 cases. Cancer 36: 1162–1168
13. Martini N, Hajdu SI, Whitmore WF, Beattie EJ (1986) Primary mediastinal germ cell tumors. Cancer 33: 763–769
14. Friedman SJ, Martin NJ (1988) Extragonadal mediastinal seminoma. Milit Med 153: 32–34
15. Jain KK, Bose GJ, Whitmore WF, Golle RS (1984) The treatment of extragonadal seminoma. J Clin Oncol 7: 820–827
16. Patcher MR, Lattes R (1964) Germinal tumors of the mediastinum: a clinico-pathologic study of adult teratomas, teratocarcinomas, choriocarcinomas and seminomas. Dis Chest 45: 301–310
17. Oberman HA, Libcke JH (1964) Malignant germinal neoplasms of the mediastinum. Cancer 17: 498–507
18. Nickels J, Franssila K (1972) Primary seminoma of the anterior mediastinum. Acta Pathol Microbiol Scand A Pathol 80: 260–262
19. Clemon GH (1983) Management of primary mediastinal seminoma. Chest 83: 263–267
20. Bell DA, Bahn AK (1987) Immunohistochemical characteristics of seminoma and its inflammatory cell infiltrate. Hum Pathol 18: 511–520
21. Levitt RG, Husbond JE, Glaser HS (1983) CT of primary germ cell tumors of the mediastinum. AJR 142: 73–78
22. Bohle A, S.U., Sonntag RW, Scheidegger JR (1986) Primary of secondary extragonadal germ cell tumors? J Urol 135: 939–943
23. Boden G, Gibb R (1951) Radiotherapy and testicular neoplasms. Lancet 2: 1195–1197
24. Cefaro GA, Luzi S, Turriziona A, Salvi G, Mermiroh L (1988) Primary mediastinal seminoma. Br J Urol 62: 461–464
25. Shem JST, Fu KH, Choi PHK, Lau WH, Khim MA, Choy D (1990) Primary mediastinal seminoma. Oncology 47: 124–127
26. Kiffer JD, Saudeman TF (1989) Primary malignant mediastinal germ cell tumors: a study of eleven cases and a review of the literature. Int J Radiat Oncol Biol Phys 17: 835–841
27. Uematsu M, Kondom, Dokiye T, Tamai S, Ando Y, Hashimoto S (1992) The role of radiotherapy in the treatment of primary mediastinal seminoma. Radiother Oncol 24: 226–230
28. Lee YM, Jackson SM (1985) Primary seminoma of the mediastinum. Cancer control agency of British Columbia experience. Cancer 55: 450–452
29. Motzer RJ, Bosl GJ, Geller NL, et al. (1988) Advanced seminoma: the role of chemotherapy and adjunction surgery. Ann Intern Med 108: 513–518
30. Giaccone G (1991) Multimodality treatment of malignant germ cell tumors of the mediastinum. Eur J Cancer 27: 273–277
31. Shultz SM, Einhorn LH, Conces DJ, Williams SD, Loehrer PJ (1989) Management of post-chemotherapy residual mass in patient with advanced seminoma: Indiana University experience. J Clin Oncol 7: 1497–1503
32. Logothetis CJ, Samuels ML, Selig DE, Dexens FH, Johnson DE, Swenson DA, von Eschenbach AC (1985) Chemotherapy of extragonadal germ cell tumors. J Clin Oncol 3: 316–325
33. Blester RJ, Lippert MC, Mills SE (1987) Late recurrence of a seminoma. J Urol 137: 749–750

8 Endocrine Tumors of the Mediastinum

THOMAS S. REEVE and LEIGH DELBRIDGE

CONTENTS

8.1 Substernal Goiter

8.1.1 Pathology

Simple goiters are thought to occur in response to any of a number of factors that impair the efficiency with which the thyroid produces its hormone. This process occurs in predisposed individuals or as the result of external factors such as iodine deficiency. Multinodular goiters subsequently develop after repeated cycles of hyperstimulation and involution. This results in both functional and anatomic heterogeneity with areas of hyperplasia, degeneration, and nodule formation within the thyroid parenchyma [1]. Thyroid tumors, either benign follicular adenoma or thyroid cancer, may arise within normal thyroid tissue or in association with a pre-existing multinodular goiter.

THOMAS S. REEVE, F.R.A.C.S., F.A.C.S., Professor Emeritus, University of Sydney, Royal North Shore Hospital, Sydney, Australia
LEIGH DELBRIDGE, M.D., F.R.A.C.S., Professor of Surgery, Endocrine Surgical Unit, Royal North Shore Hospital, Sydney, Australia

The pathologic conditions arising in a substernal goiter are identical to those occurring in a cervical thyroid gland, the only differences being in their anatomic position and subsequent clinical presentation, as well as in the potential for complications for the patient and difficulties in surgical approach.

There has been considerable discussion about the origin of substernal goiter. One possibility is that embryonic rests of thyroid tissue come to lie within the mediastinum in a substernal position, as the thyroid gland descends from the foramen caecum down through the neck during embryologic development. Nodule formation or goiter development could then occur within this ectopic thyroid tissue. A few instances of isolated mediastinal goiters have been reported [2]. It is more likely, however, that substernal goiters simply represent the downward growth through the thoracic inlet of a progressively enlarging cervical goiter. Once below the thoracic inlet, negative intrathoracic pressure further assists the downward progression of the enlarged gland. The relative loss of restriction to growth, once the bony margins of the thoracic inlet have been passed, enables the development of very large substernal components to otherwise small to moderate sized cervical goiters. In support of this concept of downward growth of large goiters is the not uncommon clinical finding, on taking a patient's history, that a previously large cervical goiter actually seemed to disappear from the neck, coinciding with the development of the retrosternal component. Other possible factors include pressure from the strap muscles or sternomastoid, pushing the enlarging goiter down into the thorax.

Further evidence for this concept can be found in the anatomic distribution of the entire blood supply of substernal goiters. Even massive goiters extending below the aortic arch are normally supplied by cervical vessels (the superior thyroid coming from the external carotid and the inferior thyroid arising from the thyrocervical trunk). The substernal component of the goiter lying within its pseudocapsule generally has no vascular connection with the major thoracic vessels with which it is in direct apposition except when a thyroideaima artery is present. The major exception to this is with true ectopic or aberrant goiters, when the blood supply may arise from the aorta, internal mammary arteries, or subclavian vessels [3].

A substernal goiter has been reported to be present in between 1% and 15% of thyroids undergoing surgery [2]. The disparity in reported incidence relates to the accuracy of the definition of a substernal component, as well as to geographic differences in the nature of thyroid disease and the incidence of nodular goiter. Indeed, in one of the earliest studies on surgery for substernal and intrathoracic goiter from the Mayo Clinic, PEMBERTON [4] attempted to define accurately the difference between substernal and true intrathoracic goiters on the basis of the extent of downward projection. Clinically, however, this is very variable, and we prefer to define substernal goiter simply as any goiter extending below the manubrium sterni with the neck extended. On this basis the incidence of substernal goiter would appear to be even higher than generally reported. In a consecutive series of 5205 thyroid operations performed in our unit over a 15-year period, 1003 had an identifiable substernal component noted either on preoperative investigation or at operation, an incidence of 19%.

8.1.2 Presentation

Many substernal goiters are asymptomatic and present incidentally, such as on a routine chest x-ray, following mass screening for tuberculosis [5, 6], or during investigation of other thoracic conditions, or even during surgical procedures such as cardiac bypass grafting [7]. A significant percentage will also be noted during surgery for a cervical goiter when an unsuspected substernal component is delivered along with the cervical goiter. Symptomatic presentation relates to the particular intrathoracic organ which happens to be compressed by the enlarging goiter. Most common are symptoms related to tracheal pressure, or compression, such as choking and dyspnea. Untreated, these may progress to complete respiratory obstruction requiring emergency surgery, especially if associated with a bleed into an intrathoracic nodule causing increased pressure within the confines of the bony boundaries of the thoracic inlet. Esophageal pressure will cause dysphagia or even full-thickness erosion and hematemesis [8], while compression of

the superior vena cava will cause venous congestion of the head and neck as well as distension of the superficial veins over the sternum and anterior chest wall (Fig. 8.1). Less common presentations arise from pressure on nerves, including voice changes associated with recurrent laryngeal nerve neuropraxia. Respiratory problems following phrenic nerve pressure, including a case of bilateral phrenic nerve palsy, have also been reported [9].

Malignancy arising in a substernal goiter will most commonly present with similar compressive symptoms, although the onset may be more rapid. Occasionally such a malignancy will present with distant metastases or local cervical nodal metastases. Anaplastic carcinoma should be suspected in the elderly with large, rapidly expanding substernal goiters. The incidence of malignancy varies considerably, with 71 patients (7%) having malignancy detected on final histology in our own series. This number, however, included incidental occult papillary carcinoma, a condition of little clinical significance in this group.

8.1.3 Investigation

Many retrosternal goiters will be detected on routine chest x-ray, although significant substernal goiters can be missed or their size underestimated when chest x-rays are relied on as the sole technique for monitoring goiter size [10]. One of the most

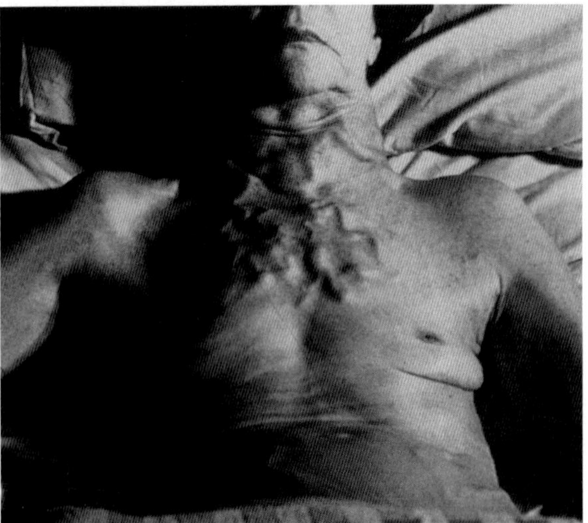

Fig. 8.1. Distension of the superficial veins over the sternum and chest wall in association with a substernal goiter causing superior vena cava obstruction

accurate radiologic signs is displacement or narrowing of the tracheal lumen. The most accurate investigation for substernal goiter, however, is a CT scan of the neck and upper mediastinum [11], and this has become the gold standard for diagnosing this form of thyroid pathology. This will display the full extent of the substernal component of the goiter, as well as the degree of involvement or compression of surrounding thoracic structures (Fig. 8.2). Magnetic resonance imaging (MRI) is as accurate as computed tomographic (CT) scanning in demonstrating upper mediastinal structures [12] but, as it has no specific advantage, it is not recommended due to the higher cost. Ultrasound will not demonstrate the substernal component and nuclear scanning is often unhelpful, as only the cervical component of very large substernal goiters will take up the isotope in more than 50% of cases [10].

Other investigations which may be of value are measurement of peak expiratory flow rate (PEFR), which some authors claim to be a sensitive index of tracheal compression [13]. It must be appreciated, however, that very marked tracheal compressive symptoms (e.g., a sensation of choking) can occur in the absence of luminal narrowing. This results from either external pressure or interruption to laminar flow with angulation of the trachea or compression of the membranous component. For this reason a normal PEFR measurement should not be used as a reason to delay or defer surgery. Patients may in fact present initially with acute airway distress requiring tracheostomy or semiurgent surgery [14].

Fine-needle aspiration biopsy, although the mainstay of investigation for cervical goiters [15], is not generally recommended for substernal goiters due to difficulties in the placement of the needle tip [7], as well as the risk of complications.

Other investigations recommended include thyroid function tests, as subclinical thyrotoxicosis is very common with large substernal goiters, especially in elderly patients. This is often unsuspected, or may present as cardiac disease [16]. Untreated, however, it could lead to major anesthetic problems. The other investigation recommended is a routine laryngeal examination for assessment of vocal cord function in order to exclude an unsuspected, asymptomatic, preexisting vocal cord palsy.

8.1.4 Management

Surgical removal is the only effective form of treatment for substernal goiter. Thyroxine suppression has not proved to be of value in attempting to shrink the size of large established nodular goiters [1] and its use is not recommended. While there is no question as to whether or not a symptomatic substernal goiter should be removed, considerable discussion surrounds the question of whether an asymptomatic, incidentally discovered, substernal goiter requires removal. Those favoring routine removal in otherwise fit patients cite the incidence of malignancy documented in such goiters (more than 20% if incidental papillary carcinomas are included), as well as the risk of sudden compression from a bleed [7]. The natural history of multinodular goiter is a slow progressive increase in size, and so it is likely that compressive symptoms will ultimately

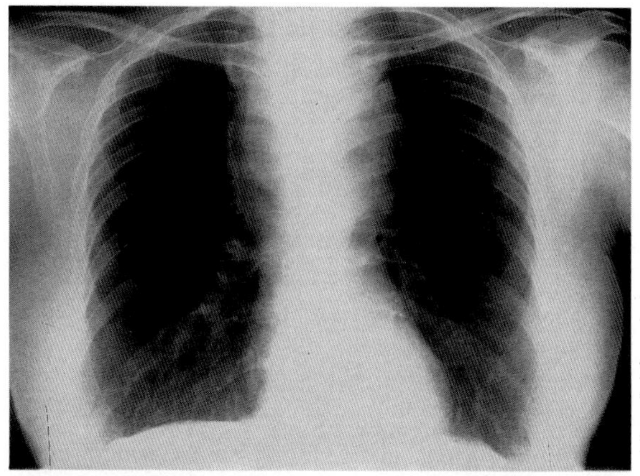

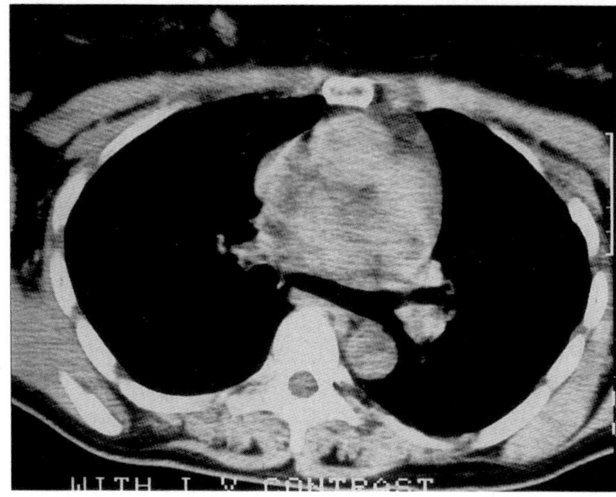

Fig. 8.2a, b. Chest x-ray (**a**) and CT scan (**b**) demonstrating compression of trachea and left main bronchus. Despite the large size, this goiter was readily removed through a cervical incision. This was achieved because although there was significant compression of intrathoracic structures, the vascular supply arose from cervical vessels

develop, should the patient live long enough. Delayed surgery for a larger substernal goiter in an older patient clearly has a higher morbidity than elective removal performed earlier. It is certainly the policy in our unit, as in many others [17], that the presence of a substernal goiter in an asymptomatic, otherwise fit patient is an indication for surgery.

Thyrotoxicosis, if present, must be treated with antithyroid agents, and the patient rendered euthyroid both clinically and biochemically before surgery is attempted.

The surgical approach to the substernal goiter should be via a standard cervical thyroidectomy incision. The vast majority of these tumors can be delivered into the neck and removed cervically. A median sternotomy is only rarely required, more frequently when the patient has had previous thyroid surgery, destroying normal tissue planes. In our own series of 1007 successive thyroidectomies for substernal goiter, a median sternotomy only had to be performed four times to achieve removal of the gland (0.4%). The surgical approach involves dividing the upper pole vessels and the middle thyroid vein in order to gain access to the prevertebral plane. Using the finger as a dissecting instrument, mobilization of the entire substernal component can usually be readily achieved, even down to below the level of the aortic arch. Once the plane inside the pseudocapsule has been mobilized, gentle traction will deliver the substernal component into the neck, where a standard subcapsular thyroidectomy can be completed. Techniques such as morcelation or the use of a sterile spoon or goiter extractor [18] should not generally be required. It can be seen in Fig. 8.2 that even very large intrathoracic goiters with marked compression of the surrounding structures can be successfully delivered into the neck. The only limiting factor is the relative sizes of the goiter and the thoracic inlet.

Where there is bilateral involvement with nodular disease, we prefer to perform a total thyroidectomy, thus avoiding the possibility of local recurrence [19]. Others advocate a subtotal procedure, with thyroxine suppression of the remnant [7]. If there is unilateral involvement, a lobectomy should be sufficient. The presence of thyroid malignancy requires a total thyroidectomy, in order to allow postoperative radioiodine ablation. The only exception is for thyroid lymphoma, where all that is required is a biopsy for tissue diagnosis. Extensive surgical removal of lymphoma of the thyroid offers no survival advantage over chemotherapy and radiotherapy [20].

Complications of surgery, including recurrent laryngeal nerve palsy and permanent hypoparathyroidism, should be less than 1% for elective surgery, when performed by the capsular technique [21].

Some authors have suggested a thoracic approach, with a lateral thoracotomy for large mediastinal goiters [22]. We believe that this is not appropriate, as there is no access to the cervical paratracheal region, where the goiter arises and where the potential for damage to recurrent nerves and parathyroid glands is highest. In addition, either a median sternotomy or a lateral thoracotomy adds a significant dimension to what is otherwise straightforward surgery.

8.2 Mediastinal Parathyroid Tumors

8.2.1 Pathology

Mediastinal parathyroid tumors are of particular historical interest in endocrine surgery. The very first patient operated on in the United States for hyperparathyroidism, a Captain Charles Martel, underwent six negative neck explorations before a 3-cm parathyroid adenoma was successfully retrieved from the mediastinum in 1932 [23]. Mediastinal parathyroid tumors either arise in ectopically located parathyroid glands or migrate into the mediastinum as they increase in size.

The superior parathyroid glands are derived from the fourth branchial pouch and are generally constant in position, being found in association with the lateral lobes of the thyroid. Movement of the pharynx and larynx with deglutition, negative intrathoracic pressure, and gravitational forces may contribute to the movement of an enlarged superior gland into the mediastinum [24]. As a result, superior gland adenomas will often be found in the posterior superior mediastinum, lying close to the esophagus, as shown by THOMPSON [25] in Fig. 8.3.

The inferior glands, on the other hand, arise from the third branchial pouch and migrate a long distance, in association with the thymus. They are generally found at the lower pole of the thyroid in the thyrothymic tract, but may occur anywhere within the anterior mediastinum. Tumors can then develop in these already ectopically placed glands. Thus inferior gland adenomas are often located within the anterior mediastinum (Fig. 8.3).

Occasionally "middle mediastinal" parathyroid adenomas have been described arising in the aorto-

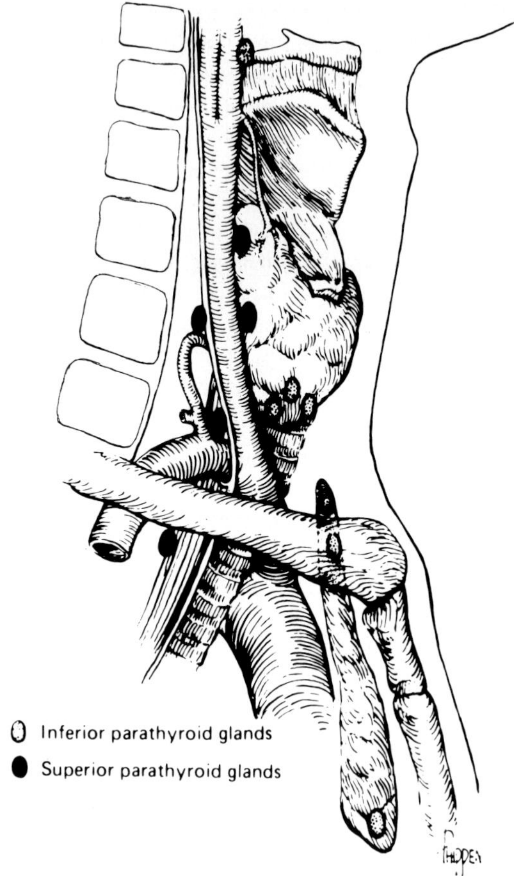

Fig. 8.3. Demonstration of the location of mediastinal parathyroid adenomas. Superior glands migrate into the posterior superior mediastinum, usually behind the esophagus, while inferior glands are found in the anterior mediastinum in association with the thymus. (From [25])

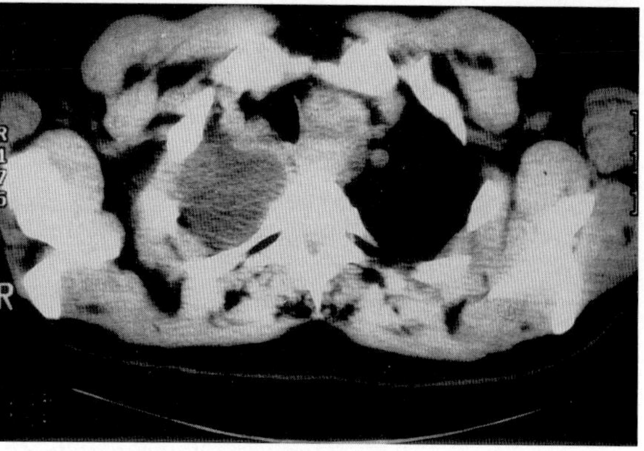

Fig. 8.4. CT scan of large double parathyroid adenomas in the posterior superior mediastinum. A median sternotomy was required to deliver the right parathyroid adenoma into the neck as its diameter exceeded the space available in the thoracic inlet. On delivery, dissection and removal was able to be performed via the cervical incision. (From 31]).

pulmonary window [26]. These may have a local blood supply, e.g., a branch from the internal mammary artery, and thus their embryologic origin is not entirely clear [25].

Primary hyperparathyroidism is most commonly due to a single parathyroid adenoma, although multiple gland disease occurs in up to 13% of cases [27]. True hyperplasia of all four glands is less common and may occur in association with one of the multiple endocrine neoplasia syndromes. Supernumerary glands (five or six or more) have been found in more than 6% of autopsy series [28, 29].

8.2.2 Presentation

Hyperparathyroidism may present with one of the classic symptoms of renal stones, bone disease, or abdominal or neuropsychiatric symptoms. An increasing number of patients nowadays present with asymptomatic hyperparathyroidism on the basis of biochemical screening studies. It is generally recommended that patients with asymptomatic hyperparathyroidism should undergo surgery in order to normalize their serum calcium levels [30].

Mediastinal parathyroid tumors will present most commonly as an incidental finding during routine cervical exploration, where a tumor is delivered into the cervical incision after exploration of the upper mediastinum. The other principal presentation is after failed initial cervical exploration, where subsequent localization studies have demonstrated the missing tumor to lie within the mediastinum. Very occasionally, the tumor may reach sufficient size to present with local compressive symptoms, or to be demonstrated on a chest x-ray or CT scan (Fig. 8.4) [31], but this is the exception, as most tumors are less than 1–2 cm in size.

8.2.3 Investigation

The only investigations required to confirm the diagnosis in the vast majority of cases of primary hyperparathyroidism are an elevated serum calcium level in the presence of an inappropriately elevated serum parathyroid hormone level when measured with a reliable whole molecule assay. Prior to an initial neck exploration, no localization studies are indicated, unless a unilateral neck exploration is planned [32]. Patients who have had a previous failed cervical exploration, however, require full localization, in an attempt to find the tumor. The initial investigation should be a CT scan of the upper mediastinum and neck. If positive, no further tests are required. If this fails to demonstrate the lesion, however, other investigations such as ultrasound, MRI, thallium or technetium scintigraphy, arteriography, and selective venous sampling have been advocated [33].

8.2.4 Management

Mediastinal parathyroid tumors are best removed surgically, although there has recently been support for angiographic ablation by embolization of mediastinal parathyroid tumors demonstrated on arteriography following failed initial cervical exploration [34].

During an initial cervical exploration, if a parathyroid gland is missing from the neck, or if the patient has parathyroid hyperplasia, the thymus is removed from the anterior mediastinum by cervical thymectomy, using blunt dissection and traction [35]. The major danger of this approach is incomplete removal, or breaking the thymus in the middle, thus leaving a parathyroid tumor which may have been at the inferior tip of the thymus, lying isolated in the anterior mediastinum. In a reoperative situation, a cervical thymectomy may be attempted, but this is often unsuccessful due to scar tissue, and so median sternotomy will be required in order to gain access to the anterior mediastinum to remove a missing inferior gland.

Superior glands lying within the posterior mediastinum can almost always be delivered into the cervical incision with blunt dissection and gentle traction. Only rarely will a thoracic incision be required for larger tumors. Middle mediastinal tumors, lying in the aortopulmonary window, generally can be approached via a median sternotomy.

8.3 Extra-adrenal Pheochromocytoma

8.3.1 Pathology

Pheochromocytomas are catecholamine-producing tumors derived from chromaffin cells. They are most commonly solitary and approximately 90% arise from within the adrenal medulla [36]. The remaining 10% are found in extra-adrenal sites, including the thorax. As most of these tumors arise in the vicinity of the sympathetic ganglia, the most common location within the thorax is in the posterior medi-

astinum, in the paravertebral gutter; however, other sites, including intrapericardial locations, have been described [37]. Most pheochromocytomas are benign although up to 10% follow a malignant course, developing local recurrence or metastases at a later date. It is frequently not possible to predict clinical course on the basis of histology of the primary tumor, which may appear benign [38, 39].

Pheochromocytoma may be familial or associated with one of the multiple endocrine neoplasia (MEN) syndromes, such as MEN IIa, where they occur in association with medullary carcinoma of the thyroid and hyperparathyroidism.

Ganglioneuromas, a neurogenic tumor seen in children, occur most frequently in the posterior mediastinum, since they also derive from the sympathetic chain [40]. Occasionally, like pheochromocytoma, they may be associated with excessive secretion of catecholamines [36].

8.3.2 Presentation

Although pheochromocytomas are rare, they represent an important curable cause of hypertension. Most present with varying combinations of the classic symptoms of paroxysmal or sustained hypertension, headache, sweating, and palpitations [41], although up to one-third may be asymptomatic and discovered incidentally or not diagnosed at all in life.

Mediastinal extra-adrenal pheochromocytomas are most commonly diagnosed after the presence of a pheochromocytoma has been confirmed biochemically but imaging studies have failed to demonstrate any abnormality in either adrenal gland. The second most common presentation is the incidental discovery of a posterior mediastinal mass on radiology of the chest.

8.3.3 Investigation

The diagnosis of pheochromocytoma is confirmed by the demonstration of elevated urinary or serum levels of catecholamines, including epinephrine, norepinephrine, and dopamine. Tumor localization is generally achieved with CT scanning, although both MRI and ^{131}I-metaiodobenzylguanidine scintigraphy are highly specific for pheochromocytoma. The T2-weighted images of pheochromocytoma are hyperdense on MRI. ^{131}I-MIBG scintigraphy is particularly useful in identifying extra-adrenal sites of pheochromocytoma due to its high specificity for that tumor [42]. Invasive techniques such as arteriography and selective venous sampling, as well as having potential major morbidity in unblocked patients, should rarely be necessary for localization nowadays.

8.3.4 Management

Surgical excision is the only form of definitive treatment for pheochromocytoma. The workup and preparation of these patients require close cooperation between surgeon, endocrinologist, and anesthesiologist. These procedures should only be performed in centres which have experience in their management [36].

The mainstay of preoperative preparation is α-blockade with an agent such as phenoxybenzamine for at least 2 weeks, to allow restoration of plasma volume. β-Blockade may be required for persistent symptoms. During surgery, close monitoring and the immediate capacity to respond to paroxysmal fluctuations in blood pressure or arrhythmias arising in association with tumor manipulation are required.

Tumors in the posterior mediastinum are best approached by a posterolateral thoracotomy whereas intrapericardial pheochromocytomas may require median sternotomy and cardiopulmonary bypass to achieve removal [37].

8.4 Thymic Carcinoid in the Multiple Endocrine Neoplasia Syndrome Type I

The multiple endocrine neoplasia syndrome type I (MEN I) is a familial syndrome which has been characterized by the presence of hyperparathyroidism, pituitary tumors and pancreatic islet cell tumors. It has recently been recognized that thymic carcinoids are another frequent feature of this syndrome, at least in some family groups. The largest known kindred in the world of such patients is found on the island state of Tasmania, Australia, and comprises more than 2000 documented members [43]. The most common cause of death in this group, rather than being peptic ulcer disease as is generally believed, has been neoplasia including thymic carcinoids in males. The other tumors causing death are bronchial carcinoids in females, pituitary tumors, malignant neuroendocrine tumors of the pancreas and adrenal carcinoma [44].

It is now recommended that routine cervical thymectomy be performed at the time of parathyroid surgery in patients suffering from MEN I and hyperparathyroidism. Not only will this remove ectopic sites of parathyroid tissue, but may also remove the potential for subsequent development of malignant thymic carcinoids.

References

1. Larsen PR, Ingbar SH (1991) The thyroid gland. In: Wilson JD, Foster DW (eds) Williams textbook of endocrinology, 8th edn. Saunders, Philadelphia, pp 357–488
2. Shahian DM (1991) Surgical treatment of intrathoracic goiter. In: Cady B, Rossi RL (eds) Surgery of the thyroid and parathyroid glands. 3rd edn. Saunders, Philadelphia, pp 215–222
3. Katlic MR, Wang CA, Grillo HC (1985) Substernal goiter. Ann Thorac Surg 39: 391–399
4. Pemberton J deJ (1921) Surgery of substernal and intrathoracic goiters. Arch Surg 2: 1–25
5. Reeve TS, Rubenstein C, Rundle FF (1957) Intrathoracic goitre: it prevalence in Sydney metropolitan mass X-ray surveys. Med J Aust 2: 149–153
6. Reeve TS, Rundle FF, Hales IB, et al. (1962) The investigation and management of intrathoracic goiter. Surg Gynec Obstet 115: 223–229
7. Snaders LA, Rossi RL, Shahian DM, Williamson WA (1992) Mediastinal goiters: the need for an aggressive approach. Arch Surg 127: 609–612
8. Parker DR, el-Shaboury AH (1992) Fatal haematemesis due to a benign retrosternal goitre. Postgrad Med J 68: 756–757
9. Manning PB, Thompson NW (1989) Bilateral phrenic nerve palsy associated with benign thyroid goiter. Acta Chir Scand 155: 429–431
10. Cohen O, Herskovitz P, Shindell B, Leiba S, Hadar H (1992) Pitfalls in the follow-up of cervical and mediastinal goiters: role of CT imaging J Laryngol Otol 106: 65–70
11. Michel LA, Bradpiece HA (1988) Surgical management of substernal goitre. Br J Surg 75: 565–569
12. Roher HD, Goretzki PE, Wahl RA, Frilling A (1989) Intrathorakale struma. Chirurg 60: 384–390
13. Stephenson BM, Shandall AA, Griffith GH (1991) Peak expiratory flow in the detection of retrosternal goitre. Ann R Coll Surg Engl 73: 215–218
14. Shaha AR, Burnett C, Alfonso A, Jaffe BM (1989) Goiters and airway problems. Am J Surg 158: 378–380
15. Reeve TS, Delbridge L, Sloan D, Crummer P (1986) The impact of fine needle aspiration biopsy on surgery for single thyroid nodules. Med J Aust 145: 308–311
16. Reeve TS, Delbridge L, Crummer P (1987) Thyroid surgery in the elderly. Ann Acad Med Singapore 16: 55–57
17. Allo MD, Thompson NW (1983) Rationale for the operative management of substernal goiters. Surgery 94: 969–977
18. Sacre R (1984) A new instrument: the goiter extractor. Head Neck 6: 1059–1060
19. Reeve TS, Delbridge L, Cohen A, Crummer P (1987)

Total thyroidectomy: the preferred option for multinodular goiter. Ann Surg 206: 782–785

20. Pyke CM, Grant CS, Habermann TM, et al. (1992) Non-Hodgkin's lymphoma of the thyroid: is more than biopsy necessary? World J Surg 16: 604–610

21. Delbridge L, Reeve TS, Khadra M, Poole AG (1992) Total thyroidectomy: the technique of capsular dissection. Aust N Z J Surg 62: 96–99

22. Waldron D, Coffey J, Murphy S, Bresnihan E, Finnegan P, Lynch V (1990) Retrotracheal goiter: a diagnostic and therapeutic problem. Ann Thorac Surg 50: 133–135

23. Cope O (1966) The story of hyperparathyroidism at the Massachussetts General Hospital. N Engl J Med 274: 1174–1185

24. Wang CA, Gaz RD, Moncure AC (1986) Mediastinal parathyroid exploration: a clinical and pathological study of 47 cases. World J Surg 10: 687–695

25. Thompson NW (1986) Surgical anatomy of hyperparathyroidism. In: Rothmund M, Wells SA (eds) Progress in surgery vol 18. Parathyroid Surgery, Karger, Basel, pp 59–79

26. Curley I, Wheeler M, Thompson NW, Grant C (1988) Challenge of the middle mediastinal parathyroid. World J Surg 12: 818–824

27. Proye CAG, Carnaille B, Bizard JP, Quievreux JL, Lecomte-Houcke M (1992) Multiglandular disease in seemingly sporadic primary hyperparathyroidism revisited: where are we in the early 1990's? A plea against unilateral exploration. Surgery 112: 1118–1122

28. Gilmour JR (1938) The gross anatomy of the parathyroid glands. J Pathol 46: 133–149

29. Akerstrom G, Malmaeus J, Bergstrom R (1984) Surgical anatomy of human parathyroid glands. Surgery 95: 14–21

30. Proceedings of the NIH consensus development conference on diagnosis and management of asymptomatic primary hyperparathyroidism: consensus development conference statement (1991) J Bone Miner Res 6 (suppl 2): 9–13

31. Fahey TJ, Hibbert E, Stiel J, Brady L, Delbridge L (1995) Giant double parathyroid adenomas presenting as hypercalcaemic crisis. Aust N Z J Surg 65: 114–115

32. Duh QY, Uden P, Clark OH (1992) Unilateral neck exploration for primary hyperparathyroidism: analysis of a controversy using a mathematical model. World J Surg 16: 654–662

33. Miller DL (1991) Pre-operative localization and interventional treatment of parathyroid tumours: when and how? World J Surg 15: 706–715

34. Doherty GM, Doppman JL, Miller DL, et al. (1992) Results of a multidisciplinary strategy for managment of mediastinal parathyroid adenoma as a cause of persistent primary hyperparathyroidism. Ann Surg 215: 101–106

35. Thomas FT (1982) Thymectomy. In: Dudley H, Pories WJ (eds) Rob & Smith's operative surgery, 4th edn. Butterworth, London, pp 387–396

36. Landsberg L, Young JB (1991) Catecholamines and the adrenal medulla. In: Wilson JD, Foster DW (eds) Williams textbook of endocrinology, 8th edn. Saunders, Philadelphia, pp 621–705

37. Saad MF, Frazier OH, Hickey RC, Samaan NA (1983) Intrapericardial pheochromocytoma. Am J Med 75: 371–375

38. van Heerden JA, Roland CF, Carney A, Sheps SG, Grant CS (1990) Long-term evaluation following resection of apparently benign pheochromocytoma(s)/paraganglioma(s) World J Surg 14: 325–329

39. Cope C, Delbridge L, Philips J, Friedlander M (1991) Prognostic significance of nuclear DNA content in phaeochromocytoma. Aust N Z J Surg 61: 695–698

40. Whittaker LD, Lynn HB (1973) Mediastinal tumours and cysts in the pediatric patient. Surg Clin North 53: 893–903

41. Gough IR, Thompson NW (1988) Phaeochromocytoma. Aust N Z J Surg 58: 365–368

42. Thompson NW, Allo MD, Shapiro B, Sisson JC, Beierwaltes WH (1984) Extra-adrenal metastatic pheochromocytoma: the role to ^{131}I-meta-iodobenzylguanidine in localization and management. World J Surg 8: 605–611

43. Shepherd JJ (1991) The natural history of multiple endocrine neoplasia type I. Arch Surg 126: 935–952

44. Wilkinson S, Teh BT, Davey KR, McArdle JP, Young M, Shepherd JJ (1993) Cause of death in multiple endocrine neoplasia. Arch Surg 128: 683–690

9 Mediastinal Paragangliomas

ROBERT B. LEE and JOSEPH I. MILLER, JR.

CONTENTS

9.1 Introduction

Paragangliomas, and particularly pheochromocytoma, have been the subject of great curiosity for some physicians and a true obsession for others. Despite the relative rarity of this tumor, it has spawned intense research into its origins, physiology, diagnosis, and treatment. Paraganglionic tumors arise from cells originating in neuroectoderm, specifically the neural crest. They may be found anywhere along the paraganglionic system from the pelvis to the cervical region (Fig. 9.1). There has been considerable confusion in the literature regarding nomenclature. In the following discussion the term "pheochromocytoma" will be used to denote chromaffin-positive paraganglioma, and "chemodectoma" will be used to describe chromaffin-negative paraganglioma. Pheochromocytomas generally are

ROBERT B. LEE, M.D., Assistant Professor of Surgery (Cardiothoracic), The Emory Clinic, 1365 Clifton Rd. NE, Atlanta, GA 30322, USA
JOSEPH I. MILLER JR., M.D., Professor of Surgery, Division of Thoracic Surgery, The Emory Clinic, 25 Prescott Street, Suite 3417, Atlanta, GA 30308, USA

functional secreting tumors while chemodectomas are not. The discussion will be limited to the occurrence in the mediastinum. Embryology, diagnosis, and management will be considered. Neurogenic tumors are the most common primary mediastinal tumor, accounting for 21% of mediastinal tumors in the adult population. The majority of these are neurilemmomas (40%–60%), ganglioneuromas and neuroblastomas (33%), and neurofibromas (10%) [1, 2]. Paragangliomas are rare. Intra-thoracic pheocychromas account for less than 1% of the total reported pheochromocytomas [3–5]. These tumors are found along the para-vertebral sulci, described by SHIELDS [6] as the costovertebral region, a potential space found along each side of the vertebral bodies and adjacent ribs. The non functioning paraganglioma or chemodectoma is likewise rare (it occurs most frequently in the middle mediastinum, e.g., cardiac chambers, pericardium, and aortic root). These tumors are found more often in adults.

The diagnosis, preoperative management, intraoperative management, and postoperative care are highly challenging. This challenge is best met by a multidisciplinary team consisting of thoracic surgeons, endocrinologists, radiologists, pathologists, and anesthesiologists. The approach will be outlined.

9.2 Historical Aspects

FRANKEL found bilateral adrenal tumors at autopsy in an 18-year-old girl who collapsed suddenly and died in 1886 [7]. Descriptions of similar clinical scenarios and autopsy findings prior to this were poor and not well documented; therefore, Frankel is generally given credit for describing the first pheochromocytoma.

MILLER reported the first intrathoracic pheochromocytoma as an incidental finding at autopsy in a 39-year-old female in 1924 [8]. The first successfully operated case of intrathoracic pheochromocytoma was reported by MAIER in 1949 [9].

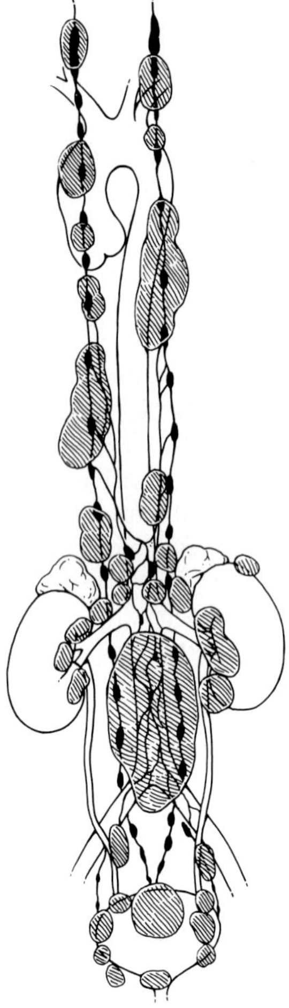

Fig. 9.1. The normal newborn paraganglionic chain is shown in *black*. The *lined areas* represent sites of extra-adrenal pheochromocytomas reported in the literature

Historical reviews of intrathoracic pheochromocytoma have previously been reported [4, 10, 11].

9.3 Histopathology and Nomenclature

9.3.1 Histology

The histologic study of the paraganglionic tumors began early when MANASSE revealed that the then unknown tumor (later to be called pheochromocytoma) was composed of cells with a staining affinity for bichromate salts [12]. These "chromaffin-positive" cells were later found to have neuro-secretory granules containing catecholamines, specifically epinephrine, while the "chromaffin-negative" cells were void of such granules. The paraganglia are composed of two predominant cell types: (a) "chief" cells similar to those of the adrenal medulla and (b) sustentacular cells similar to the satellite cells of the autonomic ganglion. The reader is referred to a standard textbook of histology or the textbook *Mediastinal Surgery* [5] for greater detail regarding histology.

9.3.2 Nomenclature

The nomenclature of these tumors has been based on location, function, and histologic staining characteristics. Thus, there were "positive chromium" tumors and "negative chromium" tumors. As the functional capabilities of the tumors were discovered, they were termed catecholamine-secreting and non-catecholamine-secreting tumors. When the relationship and similarity to the catecholamine-secreting adrenomedullary tumors or "pheochromocytoma" were recognized, it became necessary to denote their extra-adrenal location by applying the term "extra-adrenal pheochromocytomas" or "functioning paragangliomas." The nonsecreting extra-adrenal lesions are termed "nonfunctioning paragangliomas" or simply "paragangliomas." To confuse the issue further, many tumors were given names according to location: aortic body tumors, glomus jugulare, and cardiac chemodectomas.

We agree with SHAPIRO et al. [13] that the clearest and most precise terminology is "functioning paraganglioma" and "non-functioning paraganglioma." However, we acknowledge that the terms "extra-adrenal pheochromocytoma" and "chemodectoma" are the popular terms in the literature and, therefore, have accepted "functional paraganglioma" to be synonymous with "extra-adrenal pheochromocytoma" and "nonfunctioning paraganglioma" to be synonymous with "chemodectoma."

9.4 Diagnosis

Diagnosis of paraganglionic tumors of the mediastinum is based on clinical presentation, radiologic evaluation, bio-chemical analysis, and radioimmunologic localization. The development and clinical usage of the sympathetic tissue-seeking radiopharmaceutical ^{131}I-metaiodobenzylguanadine (MIBG) has revolutionized the localization [13–15] and even the treatment [15, 16] of intra-thoracic pheochromocytoma. This contribution by Shapiro and others at the University of Michigan is undoubtedly the most significant advance in the care of patients with intrathoracic pheochromocytoma in the twentieth century. The clinical presentation, radiologic modalities, and use of ^{131}I-MIBG will be discussed.

9.4.1 Clinical Presentation

The presentation of functioning paraganglioma (pheochromocytoma) is a manifestation of its elaboration of catecholamines. The presentation of non-functioning paraganglioma (chemodectoma) is most often due to the tumor's space-occupying nature and compression or invasion of local structures. As stated previously, the actual incidence of paraganglionic tumors remains elusive as many are not diagnosed until autopsy [11]. Between 0.1% and 0.5% of newly diagnosed hypertensives are found to have pheochromocytoma, and only 1%–2% are eventually found to have an intrathoracic location of their tumor. Of this relatively small number, 80% are found in the paravertebral sulci arising from the aortosympathetic ganglia. The peak incidence occurs between ages 30 and 40 years. The sexes are equally affected [17].

The functioning chromaffin-positive paragangliomas (pheochromocytoma) may present with mild symptoms or as the classic pheochromocytoma syndrome. The symptoms are a function of the norepinephrine-secreting attributes of the tumor: hypertension, hypermetabolism, and glucose intolerance. The non-secreting paragangliomas (chemodectoma) present due to mass effect and local pressure effects. Due to their nonsecretory nature they frequently are of considerable size at the time of presentation, often being found incidentally on routine chest x-rays [18]. Intrathoracic paraganglioma in the costovertebral angle may cause nerve root or spinal cord compression, lung compression, or Horner's syndrome if the sympathetic chain is compressed. Those found in the visceral compartment of the mediastinum cause venous compression initially and, if allowed to persist untreated, may cause arterial compression. Tumors found in an intracardiac location may cause conduction system dysfunction or obliteration of the cardiac chambers [14, 19–21].

9.4.2 Biochemical Diagnosis

The presence of a previously undiagnosed mediastinal mass and malignant hypertension should prompt one to suspect the possibility of an intra-thoracic pheochromocytoma. A chemical analysis of the plasma and urinary catecholamines was one of the earliest methods of detection. It remains an important screening tool for the patient in whom pheochromocytoma is suspected. Sensitivity and specificity are related to the collection of the specimen and the expertise of the laboratory conducting the study.

Serum plasma levels of epinephrine, norepinephrine, and dopamine can be fractionated from the total serum catecholamines. These levels are extremely labile and great care must be taken to avoid drug interference and stimulation or stress during collection. Samples must be collected from an indwelling intravenous catheter placed 30–60 min before sampling begins in an unstressed, hydrated, supine patient. Values may vary between laboratories. Elevation of catecholamines and plasma should be confirmed by analysis of urine samples [10].

Vanillylmandelic acid (VMA) is the chief urinary metabolite of epinephrine and norepinephrine. It can be collected as a 2-, 12-, or 24-h specimen. The 24-h collections are affected less by transient changes. Patients should be placed on a special diet prior to collection of the specimen to avoid the influence of dietary phenolic acids and vanillin. The normal 24-h range for VMA is between 2 and 9 mg. A urinary epinephrine level of > 50 μg and a norepinephrine level > 150 μg will establish the diagnosis in $> 90\%$ of the patients with clinically active tumors. Marked elevation may suggest an extra-adrenal location of the tumor [5, 6, 10].

Occasionally urinary and plasma catecholamine levels are equivocal. MACDOUGALL et al. recommend the overnight clonidine suppression test as a sensitive indicator for unmasking equivocal cases of pheochromocytoma. They feel that timed collection of urinary catechols and metabolites is more reliable, cheaper, and avoids the possible labile nature of plasma measurements [22].

9.4.3 Radiologic Diagnosis

Once a patient with an intrathoracic mass and plasma catecholamine studies suggesting a pheochromocytoma or chemodectoma is identified, tumor localization ensues. It is extremely important to evaluate the entire body for the presence of other primary tumors or possible metastatic disease. Multiple modalities exists for localization: chest x-ray, esophagogram, angiography, venography, computed tomography (CT), magnetic resonance imaging (MRI), echocardiography, and ^{131}I-MIBG scintigraphy. No one modality is 100% accurate. Therefore, we, along with other authors, recommend multimodality imaging for accurate localization of the lesion in question as well as other possible tumors [23–27].

A posteroanterior and a lateral chest x-ray may provide the first indication of a mass in the case of a nonfunctioning paraganglioma. An abnormal shadow in the costovertebral angle or distortion of the atria or aorta in the cardiac silhouette may be present. Bony destruction or pulmonary metastasis may be observed on the chest x-ray. High-resolution dynamic CT has been in existence for more than 15 years. GROSS and co-workers were among the first to note that intracardiac and intrapericardial masses could be accurately and reliably imaged with the new high-resolution CT [28]. SHIN et al. describe an intrathoracic pheochromocytoma as a well-demarcated mass lesion of varying size, most of which enhances with contrast [29]. It is important to note that CT alone cannot distinguish between functioning and nonfunctioning paraganglioma. Visualization by MRI holds promise as a future enhancement modality in the diagnosis of intrathoracic pheochromocytoma but at the present time is not significantly advantageous over high-resolution CT [27].

9.4.4 Nuclear Medicine Technique

As indicated above, the development of the sympathetic tissue-seeking radiopharmaceutical ^{131}I-MIBG [16] at the University of Michigan in the early 1980s has unquestionably been the greatest step forward in the localization of pheochromocytoma to date. The technique as described by SHAPIRO et al. [16] was used in 400 patients suspected to have pheochromocytoma [13, 15]. They found the overall sensitivity to be 87.4% and the specificity, 98.9%. False-negatives do exist, usually when the tumor is intra-adrenal (10%) [26]. However, other authors have confirmed the sensitivity to be about 80% [23, 26]. This noninvasive technique has made localization safer and more accurate, almost eliminating the need for arteriography and venography [24].

9.4.5 Approach to Diagnosis and Localization

Presently we recommend that patients suspected of having an intrathoracic paraganglioma undergo mul-

timodality investigation. Those suspected of having a pheochromocytoma should have plasma levels of catecholamines assayed; if the findings are equivocal, they should then have urinary catecholamines and metabolites analyzed. A provocative test such as clonidine suppression is sometimes necessary. This should always be done in clinical investigation centers by strict protocol. ^{131}I-MIBG should then be used for screening and localization. CT should also be used to confirm the location and especially to evaluate for possible undetected intra-adrenal masses. MRI and echocardiography may be used to better define the anatomic relationship to other surrounding structures prior to resection. It may not be possible safely to obtain tissue diagnosis of the nonfunctioning paraganglioma (chemodectoma) prior to resection. We, like others [24–27], believe that ^{131}I-MIBG and CT scanning are complementary and when combined significantly increase one's ability to accurately diagnose and predict the resectability of intrathoracic paraganglioma.

9.5 Surgical Management

Surgical management remains the best option for cure of both functioning and nonfunctioning paragangliomas. A successful outcome requires thorough preoperative preparation, skilled anesthetic management, and precise expeditious surgery. Nonfunctioning paragangliomas once identified, can be safely resected depending on the anatomic location and involvement of contiguous structures. Functioning paragangliomas present a unique challenge due to their secretion of catecholamines. Therefore, many of the following comments pertain predominantly to intrathoracic pheo-chromocytomas.

9.5.1 Preoperative Preparation

Preoperative preparation includes evaluation of cardiac function, consideration of α- or β-blockade, volume replacement, and provision for transfusion requirements. Patients with long-term unopposed catecholamine secretion may develop cardiomyopathy; therefore, determination of cardiac contractility and ejection fraction is mandatory. Thallium stress test will provide this information as well as delineate areas of ischemia.

Pharmacologic management prior to resection has made surgery increasingly safe over the last decade [5, 10, 11]. Routine α-blockade with phenoxybenzamine is recommended and routinely used by some authors [5, 10, 30]. SHAPIRO recommends phenoxybenzamine be begun 1–2 weeks prior to surgery at a dose of 10 mg bid., increased every other day with the goal being normotension or near normotension with slight postural hypotension [31]. β-Blockade also may be utilized as it is helpful in avoiding supraventricular tachycardia. The preoperative preparation is generally in the hands of the endocrinologist in close consultation with his surgical colleagues. Anesthetic management can be highly complicated and discussion of this will be left to texts on anesthetic management of intrathoracic pheochromocytomas.

9.5.2 Principles of Surgical Management

The approach to and resection of intrathoracic parangangliomas are dictated by: (a) location – middle mediastinum versus posterior mediastinum – and (b) functional versus nonfunctional status (pheochromocytoma or chemodectoma). SHAPIRO and FIG state that paragangliomas found in the anterior mediastinum are usually closely associated with the thymus and extremely rare [31]. Intracaval paragangliomas are also rare but have been reported. RUTEGARD et al. reported a nonfunctioning paraganglioma arising in the superior vena cava, causing superior vena cava syndrome, which was successfully resected [32]. ORRINGER et al. have succinctly outlined the surgical principles of resection of intrathoracic paragangliomas [30] (Table 9.1). The great majority of intrathoracic paragangliomas occur in the posterior mediastinum. However, with the increased

Table 9.1. Surgical principles of resection for intrathoracic paraganglioma

1. Complete surgical excision is the only definitive curative therapy for pheochromocytoma
2. Wide surgical exposure via postero-lateral thoracotomy or median sternotomy
3. Early isolation and interruption of venous drainage to reduce systemic catecholamine release
4. Minimal tumor manipulation prior to isolation of venous drainage
5. Meticulous hemostasis
6. Removal of the tumor with capsule intact to reduce seeding of operative field (posterior mediastinal tumors)
7. Cardiac pheochromocytomas (middle mediastinum) are soft fleshy tumors, unencapsulated, and may require resection of myocardium
8. Cardiopulmonary bypass should be available

use of ^{131}I-MIBG and refinement of CT scans and MRI scans increasing numbers of middle mediastinal paragangliomas are being reported [21, 33–35].

9.5.3 Middle Mediastinal Paragangliomas

BESTERMAN is generally cited as being the first to resect a cardiac pheochromocytoma, the operation being performed on 13 May 1970 (published 1974) [36]. Almost simultaneously (on 17 June 1970), WILSON et al. [37], in Australia, resected a tumor arising from the right intra-atrial groove (published February 1974). In their paper they note that the first report was published in 1963 by PEIPER and GOLESTAN [38]. This report of a pheochromocytoma found between the left pulmonary artery and aorta is the earliest report of resection of an intrapericardial pheochromocytoma. NAGANT DE DENCHAISNES et al. reported a pheochromocytoma arising in the aorticopulmonary window in 1960 [39]. With the introduction of ^{131}I-MIBG have come numerous reports and reviews [33–35].

ORRINGER et al. state that paragangliomas of the middle mediastinum are essentially cardiac tumors arising from coronary paraganglia or visceral autonomic paraganglia of the arteries [30]. The majority arise from the left atrium [21, 30, 33–35], including the intra-atrial septum [40–42]. Two reports have noted subepicardial tumors involving coronary arteries [43, 44] and coronary sinus [45].

The intrapericardial location dictates an approach by either right or left posterolateral thoracotomy or median sternotomy. We agree with other authors [30, 34, 35] that cardiopulmonary bypass with cardioplegic arrest offers the best method of isolating the tumor from the circulation, thereby avoiding intraoperative hypertensive crisis. These tumors are highly vascular and occasionally derive their blood supply from coronary artery tributaries. They may even involve the coronary artery proper. Therefore, in totally resecting the mass it may be necessary to ligate the coronary artery, thus mandating the vessel be bypassed. When the tumor is associated with the atria, total resection may mandate repair of the atrial free wall or septum with autogenous or bovine pericardium. SHIMAYAMA et al. point out that cardiac pheochromocytomas do not behave as do their adrenal counterparts [46]. They are unencapsulated and somewhat invasive, frequently requiring full-thickness resection of atrial free wall or septum. They generally cannot be shelled out.

Nonfunctioning paragangliomas of the middle mediastinum have also been reported. It is somewhat difficult to separate cardiac paraganglioma from the more common aortic body paraganglioma. GOPALAKRISHNAN et al. reported a nonfunctioning paraganglioma (chemodectoma) of the heart involving the left ventricle. They reviewed the literature up to that time, stating that only four other chemodectomas of the heart had been previously reported [19]. Since then LEVI et al. have reported a large chemodectoma of the right ventricular outflow tract [47] and most recently (in 1991) BIRD and SEILER have reported a chemodectoma near the coronary ostia [48]. Somewhat more common are the paragangliomas arising from the supra-aortic or aorticopulmonary paraganglia. OLSON and SALYER reviewed the world literature and added four cases in their report on the subject. Thirty-nine cases of aortic body chemodectomas found in the interior mediastinum were reported [49].

9.5.4 Posterior Mediastinal Paragangliomas

Paragangliomas arising in the costovertebral area are relatively more common [50–52] and nonfunctioning tumors have been reported [18,53]. They are resected through a posterolateral thoracotomy, generally behaving more like their intra-abdominal counterparts in being much easier to resect than paragangliomas of the middle mediastinum [52]. Resection may require removal of a portion of the vertebra if the neural foramen has been invaded [52].

9.6 Management of Malignant Disease

Malignant paragangliomas, both functioning [54] and nonfunctioning [20], have been reported. Malignancy is difficult to establish histologically as both benign and malignant tumors may have necrosis and mitotic figures [20,21,55–57]. Only the presence of paraganglionic tissue in nonchromaffin tissue or distant metastasis would indicate malignancy. The rate of malignancy is approximately 10%–20% [6,20,21]. The incidence of malignancy of extra-adrenal pheochromocytomas is 20%–50% higher than that of adrenal pheochromocytomas [10, 11]. Liver, lung, and skeleton are the most frequent sites of distant metastasis. Resection of solitary metastatic pheochromocytomas or recurrent disease is indicated. Surgical debulking of unresectable lesions is indicated to make medical management easier. As SCOTT points out, long-term survival is possible and the natural course of the disease is variable [10]. Five-year mortality is approximately 45%.

Pharmacologic therapy of metastatic pheochromocytoma is directed toward management of hypertension and alleviation of pain. External beam radiation therapy of 30–60 Gy has been used for palliation of bone pain as well as control of tumors not completely resected [48, 55, 57]. It would appear that radiation therapy has a role in managing incompletely excised tumors; however, only a few cases have been reported and long-term follow-up is lacking.

Various chemotherapeutic agents have been used for treatment of metastatic pheochromocytoma, both as single agents [58] and as combination therapy [59, 60]. AVERBUCH et al. showed a complete or partial response in 8 of 14 patients (57%) treated with a combination of cyclophosphamide, vincristin, and dacarbazine [60]. Cisplatin and 5-fluorouracil were used by SRIMUNINNIMIT and WAMPLER to treat a case of familial pheochromocytoma and yielded an objective response [61].

Finally, as stated previously, ^{131}I-MIBG has been used not only to localize pheochromocytomas but also to treat metastatic disease [15]. Both THOMPSON et al. [15] and CORNFORD et al. [62] have shown ^{131}I-MIBG to be beneficial in the treatment of metastatic disease.

References

1. Davis RD, Oldham NH Jr, Sabiston DC (1987) Primary cysts and neoplasms of the mediastinum: recent changes in clinical presentation; methods of diagnosis, management, and results. Ann Thorac Surg 44: 229
2. Pearson FG (1992) Mediastinal tumors. Semin Thorac Cardiovasc Surg 4: 1
3. Gellad F, Whitley J, Shamaddin AKM (1980) Silent malignant intrathoracic pheochromocytoma. South Med J 73: 513
4. Symington T, Goodall AC (1953) Studies in pheochromocytoma. Glasgow Med J 34: 75–110
5. Shields TW (1991) Mediastinal surgery. Lea & Febiger, Philadelphia, pp 254–271
6. Shields TW (1989) General thoracic surgery, 3rd edn. Lea & Febiger, New York, pp 1096–1123
7. Frankel F (1886) Ein Fall von doppelseitigen, vollig latent verlaufenen Nebennierentumor und gleichseitigen Nephritis mit Veränderungen am Circulations – Appart und Retinitis. Arch Pathol Anat 103: 244
8. Miller JW (1924) Ein Paragangliom des Brustsympathicus. Centrall P Allg Pathol. Pathol Anat 1924; 35: 85
9. Maier HC (1949) Intrathoracic pheochromocytoma with hypertension. Ann Surg 130: 1059

10. Scott HW Jr (1990) Surgery of the adrenal glands. Lippincott, New York, pp 187–223
11. Modlin IM, Farndon JR, Shepherd A, et al. (1979) Pheochromocytoma in 72 patients: clinical and diagnostic features, treatment and long term results. Br J Surg 66: 456–465
12. Manasse P (1903) Zum Histologie and Histogenes der primären Nieateschuateles. 145: 127
13. Shapiro B, Brahm ☒, Kopp JE, Sisson JC, et al. (1985) Iodine-131 metaiodobenzylguanidine for the locating of suspected pheochromocytoma: experience in 400 cases. J Nucl Med 26: 576
14. Shapiro B, Sisson J, Kalif V (1984) The location of middle mediastinal pheochromocytoma. J Thorac Cardiovasc Surg 87: 814
15. Thompson NW, Alto MD, Shapiro B, et al. (1984) Extra-adrenal and metastatic pheochromocytoma: the role of ^{131}I-metaiodobenzylguanadine (^{131}I-MIBG) in localization and management. World J Surg 8: 605–611
16. Shapiro B, Sisson JC, Lloyd R (1984) Malignant pheochromocytoma: clinical, biochemical and scintographic characterization. Clin Endocrinol 20: 189–203
17. Freier DT, Eckhauser FE, Harrison TS (1980) Pheochromocytoma: a persistently problematic and still potentially lethal disease. Arch Surg 115: 388
18. Ashley DJ, Evans CJ (1966) Intrathoracic carotid body tumour (chemodectoma). Thorax 21: 184
19. Gopalakrishnan R, Ticzon AR, Cruz PA (1978) Cardiac paraganglioma (chemodectoma); a case report and review of the literature. J Thorac Cardiovasc Surg 76: 183–189
20. Routh A, et al. (1982) Malignant chemodectoma of the posterior mediastinum. South Med J 75: 879
21. Johnson TL et al. (1985) Cardiac paraganglioma-a clincopathologic and immunohistochemical study of four cases. Am J Surg Pathol 9: 827
22. MacDougall IC, Christopher GI, Stewart H (1988) Overnight clonidine suppression test in diagnosis and exclusion of pheochromocytoma. Am J Med 84: 993–1000
23. Sheps SG, Brown ML (1985) Localization of mediastinal paraganglioma (pheochromocytoma). Chest 87: 807
24. Bravo EL, Gifford RW (1984) Pheochromocytoma diagnosis, localization and management. N Engl J Med 311: 1298–1303
25. Francis IR, Glazier GM, Shapiro B (1983) Complementary roles of CT scanning and ^{131}I-MIBG scintigraphy in the diagnosis of pheochromocytoma. A J R 141: 719–725
26. Chatal JR, Charbonnel B (1985) Comparisons of iodobenzylguanidine imaging with computed tomography in locating pheochromocytoma. J Clin Endocrinol Metab 61: 769–772
27. Quint LE, Glazier GM, Francis IR (1987) Pheochromocytoma and paraganglioma: comparison of MR imaging with CT and I-^{131}-MIBG scintigraphy. Radiology 165: 89–93
28. Gross BH, Glazier GM, Francis IR (1983) CT of intracardiac and intrapericardial masses. A J R 140: 903–907
29. Shin MS, Gupta KL, Ho KJ (1986) Thoracic pheochromocytoma: computed tomographic characteristics. South Med J 79: 244–245
30. Orringer MB, Sisson JC, Glazier G (1985) Surgical treatment of cardiac pheochromocytoma. J Thorac Cardiovasc Surg 89: 753–757
31. Shapiro B, Fig LM (1989) Medical therapy of pheochromocytoma. In: Barkon A (ed) Medical therapy of endocrine tumors, vol 18, no. 2. Endocrinology and metabolism clinics of North America. Saunders, Philadelphia, pp 433–448
32. Rutegard J, Granstrand M, Aberg T (1992) Intracaval paraganglioma causing superior vena caval syndrome. Eur J Cardiothorac Surg 6: 337–338
33. Aravot DJ, Banner NR, Cantor AM, et al. (1992) Location, localization and surgical treatment of cardiac pheochromocytoma. Am J Cardiol 69: 283–285
34. Carval P, Chachques JC, Dervanian P (1992) Cardiac pheochromocytoma. Ann Thorac Surg 53: 356–361
35. Abad C, Jimenez P, Santana C (1992) Primary cardiac paraganglioma. J Cardiovasc Surg 33: 768–772
36. Besterman E, Bromley LL, Peart WS (1974) An intrapericardial pheochromocytoma. Br Heart J 36: 318–320
37. Wilson AC, Bennett RC, Niall JR, et al. (1974) An unusual case of intrathoracic pheochromocytoma. Aust NZ J 44: 27–32
38. Peiper HJ, Golestan C (1963) Thoraxchirurgie 10: 517–519
39. Nagant de Denchaisnes C, et al. (1960) Pheochromocytomes extra-surrenalius multiples avec "dystrophio d'Albright" et homongiones cutanes. Schweiz Med Wochenschr 33: 886–890
40. Hodgson SF, Sheps SG, Subramarnian, et al. (1984) Catecholamine-secreting paraganglia of the intra-atrial septum. Am J Med 77: 757–761
41. Kawasuji M, Matsunaga Y, Iwa T (1989) Cardiac pheochromocytoma of the intra-atrial septum. Eur J Cardiothorac Surg 3: 175–177
42. Lee HH, Brenner WI, Vardhan I, et al. (1990) Cardiac pheochromocytoma originating in the intra-atrial septum. Chest 97: 760–762
43. Rosemond TL, Hamburg MS, Vacels JL, et al. (1992) Intrapericardial pheochromocytoma. Am J Cardiol 70: 700–705
44. Orstein HH, Green GE, Kancherla PL (1984) Aortico-coronary paraganglioma, anatomic relationship of left coronary artery to paraganglia of the aorta. 84: 33–36
45. David TE, Lenker SC, Marquez JA, et al. (1986) Pheochromocytoma of the heart. Ann Thorac Surg 41: 98–100
46. Shimayama Y, Kawada K, Imamura H (1987) A functioning intrapericardial paraganglioma (pheochromocytoma). Br Heart J 57: 380–383
47. Levi B, Cain AS, Dorzab WE (1982) Coronary paraganglioma. Clin Cardiol 5: 505–510
48. Bird DJ, Seiler MW (1991) Aorticopulmonary paraganglioma (aortic body tumor) report of a case. Ultrastruct Pathol 15: 475–479
49. Olson JC, Salyer WR (1978) Mediastinal paraganglioma (aortic body tumors), a report of four cases and review of the literature. Cancer 41: 2405
50. McNeil AD, Grodin BM, Neville AM (1970) Intrathoracic pheochromocytoma. Br J Surg 57: 457–461
51. Gellad F, Whitley J, Shamsuddin AKM (1980) Silent malignant intrathoracic pheochromocytoma. South Med J 73: 513–514
52. Ogawa J, Inouri H, Kode S, et al. (1981) Functioning paraganglia in the posterior mediastinum. Ann Thorac Surg 33: 507–509
53. Enora PB, Bangioriani HL, Sgarbresi RN, et al. (1988) Non-functioning paraganglia of the posterior mediastinum. Scand J Thorac Cardiovasc Surg 22: 295–297
54. Prenot J, Schmitt M, Vicleareht M (1983) Rare forms of pheochromocytoma in children. Prog Pediatr Surg 16: 97–106
55. Assaf HM, Al-Moman AA, Martin JD (1992) Aortico-pulmonary paraganglioma. A case report with immunohistochemical studies and literature review. Arch Pathol Lab Med 116: 1085–1087

56. Pantansmitz D, Soreli P (1989) Multiple malignant paraganglioma. A case report. S Afr Med J 76: 441–443
57. Odze R, Begin LR (1990) Malignant paraganglioma of the posterior mediastinum. A case report and review of the literature. Cancer 65: 564–569
58. Feldman JM (1983) Treatment of metastatic pheochromocytoma with streptozocin. Arch Intern Med 143: 1799–1800
59. Keiser HR, Goldstein DS, Wade JC (1985) Treatment of malignant pheochromocytoma with combination chemotherapy. Hypertension 7 (suppl 1): 18–24
60. Averbuch SD, Steakley CS, Young RC, et al. (1988) Malignant pheochromocytoma: effective treatment with a combination of cyclophosphamide, vincristin, and dacarbazine. Ann Intern Med 109: 267–273
61. Srimuninnimit V, Wampler GC (1991) Case report of metastatic familial pheochromocytoma treated with cisplatin and 5–fluorouracil. Cancer Chemother Pharmacol 28: 217–219
62. Cornford EJ, Wastri ML, Morgan DA (1992) Malignant paraganglioma of the mediastinum: a further diagnostic and therapeutic use of radiolabelled mIBG. Br J Radiol 65: 75–78

10 Neurogenic Tumors of the Mediastinum

JOHN C. WAIN

CONTENTS

10.1 Introduction

Mediastinal neurogenic tumors arise from the neural elements of the peripheral, autonomic, or paraganglionic nervous systems found within the thorax. All mediastinal neurogenic tumors have an embryologic origin related to the neural crest. However, differences in predominance of specific neural cell types (nerve sheath, ganglion, or neurite) and in degrees of maturation allow for clinicopathologic classification. Neuron-specific enolase and synaptophysin, common immunohistochemical markers for neural tissue, are expressed by all of these neoplasms [1, 2].

No specific etiologic factors for neurogenic mediastinal tumors have been identified with the exception of von Recklinghausen's neurofibromatosis (NF). NF is a rare hamartomatous disorder of the ectoderm and mesoderm with a genetic pattern of inheritance demonstrating extremely variable degrees of penetrance. The disease, which may be classified into central and peripheral forms, results in multiple neurogenic tumors. The peripheral form is associated with an increased incidence of neurogenic mediastinal tumors of *all* histologic types [3]. In

JOHN C. WAIN, M.D., Assistant Professor of Surgery, Harvard Medical School; Director, Lung Transplant Program, General Thoracic Surgical Services, Massachusetts General Hospital, Boston, MA 02114, USA

addition, mediastinal neurogenic tumors found in NF are more likely to be malignant and to demonstrate intraspinal extension from the thorax [4, 5].

10.2 Incidence

Neurogenic tumors of the mediastinum are the most common mediastinal tumors in the pediatric population, accounting for 50%–60% of all mediastinal tumors. Among adults, neurogenic tumors are typically the second most common type of mediastinal tumor, accounting for 10%–35% of lesions in collected series. Presently, thymic neoplasms are identified more commonly than neurogenic neoplasms in adults, due in part to a more frequent identification of thymic tumors by computed tomographic scanning of the chest [6–7].

10.3 Classification

Mediastinal neurogenic tumors are divided into nerve sheath, autonomic, and paraganglionic subtypes based on histologic predominance of the various cellular components. Each subtype includes both benign and malignant variants (Table 10.1).

Table 10.1. Pathologic classification of mediastinal neurogenic tumors

Nerve sheath tumors
    Benign
        Neurilemmoma (benign schwannoma)
        Neurofibroma
    Malignant
        Malignant schwannoma

Autonomic nervous tumors
    Benign
        Ganglioneuroma
    Malignant
        Ganglioneuroblastoma
        Neuroblastoma

Paraganglionic tumors
    Aortic body (branchiometric) paraganglioma
    Aorticosympathetic paraganglioma

The distribution of the various neural elements within the thorax determines the location of the various subtypes. Intercostal nerves and the paravertebral sympathetic chain are the site of origin for 95% of mediastinal neurogenic tumors. Since these nerves and ganglia are concentrated in the paravertebral sulcus region, commonly designated the posterior mediastinum, this is the most common location for both nerve sheath and autonomic neurogenic tumors. Paraganglionic tumors are associated with both the posterior sympathetic chain and the middle mediastinal cardiac plexus [4, 9, 10].

10.3.1 Nerve Sheath Tumors

Nerve sheath tumors are derived from the Schwann cells surrounding neurites. They are the most common subtype of mediastinal neurogenic tumor, accounting for 40%–65% of cases in reported series. Benign variants, accounting for more than 95% of cases, include neurilemmomas (benign schwannomas) and neurofibromas. Malignant nerve sheath tumors of all types are classified as malignant schwannomas [4, 10–12].

The peak incidence of nerve sheath tumors is in the third and fourth decades. They are typically asymptomatic and have an indolent growth pattern. If symptoms do occur, they are most commonly due to neural compression in the region of the tumor or along the involved nerve trunk. Localized or neuritic pain, somatic nerve palsy (e.g., of brachial plexus branches), or cord compression due to intraspinal extension of the tumor are most likely. Rarely, compression of other intrathoracic structures may occur if the tumor is very large. Symptomatic nerve sheath tumors are more likely to be malignant schwannomas [8–10].

Neurilemmomas are the most common nerve sheath tumor. They may arise from nerves throughout the thorax, including the brachial plexus and vagus, as well as the more common intercostal nerve. Grossly, an encapsulated mass arising lateral to the underlying nerve is apparent. The tumor is firm and gray-tan on sectioning. Histologically, orderly proliferation of Schwann cells within the endoneurium, without involvement of the nerve fiber, is seen. The cells may be in a dense, palisading arrangement (Antonio type A) or a loose, myxomatous arrangement (Antonio type B). Clinical behavior does *not* correlate with the particular stromal arrangement [13].

Neurofibromas account for one-fourth of nerve sheath tumors. NF is identified in 30% of patients with neurofibromas [3, 5]. Grossly, these tumors are pseudoencapsulated and are friable and yellowish gray on sectioning. Histologically, cellular proliferation is disorderly, with fibrillary processes separated by a loose matrix. The parent nerve is involved, resulting in diffuse expansion of the nerve into a tangled network of Schwann cells mixed with axons [6, 11].

Malignant schwannomas account for less than 5% of nerve sheath tumors. The majority are associated with NF. Local invasion or distant metastases are common. Grossly, they are unencapsulated and firm. Histologically, hypercellularity with cellular palisading and mitotic figures are seen. Mitoses, however, may be widely dispersed, hampering accurate intraoperative diagnosis of these lesions [9, 13].

10.3.2 Autonomic Nervous Tumors

The second most common type of mediastinal neurogenic tumor is those tumors demonstrating autonomic nervous differentiation. These account for 35%–55% of tumors in collected series, and occur with a greater frequency in pediatric populations. Subtypes include ganglioneuroma, ganglioneuroblastoma, and neuroblastoma, each demonstrating ganglion cells mixed with a varying amount of other neural elements (Schwann cell, neurites). The subclassification of autonomic tumors incorporates differences in differentiation and biologic behavior among these neoplasms. Ganglioneuromas are well differentiated, benign lesions, while neuroblastomas are typically undifferentiated, malignant lesions. Ganglioneuroblastomas have an intermediate histologic appearance and biologic behavior.

Two-thirds of autonomic nervous tumors are found in patients less than 20 years of age [7, 13]. Malignant behavior is noted in more than one-half of cases, and the rate of growth for autonomic tumors is generally faster than for other mediastinal neurogenic tumors. Symptoms occur more frequently with these tumors than with nerve sheath tumors, correlating to both their more rapid rate of growth and their potential for production of catecholamines and other vasoactive substances by the neuroepithelial elements contained in these lesions. In addition to symptoms of neural compression, dorsal spine scoliosis, hypertension, diarrhea, and cutaneous flushing may be noted [14].

Ganglioneuromas, the benign form of autonomic nervous tumor, account for 40%–60% of these lesions. Most commonly they arise from the posterior mediastinal sympathetic chain. Grossly, they are encapsulated and, on sectioning, soft with a gray surface. Microscopically, ganglion cells, surrounded by a clear lacunar zone, intermixed with fibrillary processes separated by a loose connective tissue matrix, are seen. Myelinated and unmyelinated axons may be seen intermingled in the tumor [11].

Ganglioneuroblastomas account for 10%–15% of autonomic nervous tumors. They may be found throughout the posterior mediastinum. Grossly and histologically they may resemble neuroblastomas. Histologic evidence of ganglionic differentiation and a less aggressive clinical behavior serve to distinguish ganglioneuroblastomas [15, 16].

Neuroblastomas, the most malignant autonomic nervous tumor, account for half of mediastinal autonomic nervous neoplasms. Intrathoracic neuroblastomas represent 20% of all neuroblastomas and are more likely to present with an autoimmune syndrome of acute cerebellar ataxia, opsoclonus, and chaotic nystagmus than are extrathoracic neuroblastomas. The age of presentation of intrathoracic cases is similar to that of extrathoracic neuroblastoma, with half of all cases arising within the first 2 years of life and 90% arising by 8 years of age. Grossly, these tumors are typically large with a varying degree of capsule formation. Histologically, characteristic dark neuroepithelial cells with pseudorosette formation and foci of calcification are seen. Occasionally, glial or ganglionic differentiation is noted, and rare instances of spontaneous maturation to ganglioneuroma have been described [13, 14].

10.3.3 Paraganglionic Tumors

Paraganglionic tumors are rare mediastinal neurogenic tumors, representing less than 5% of these neoplasms in collected series. These tumors arise from paraganglionic tissue, which is normally present at various sites in the thorax, including both the middle and the posterior mediastinum. Unlike other mediastinal neurogenic tumors, paragangliomas may be found in either site with equal frequency. They are classified according to their site of origin into aortic body (branchiometric) paragangliomas, originating in the middle mediastinum, and aorticosympathetic paragangliomas, arising in the costovertebral sulcus (posterior mediastinum) [16].

Paragangliomas are histologically identical to pheochromocytomas and may be functional or nonfunctional with regard to the production of catecholamine and other vasoactive substances. They tend to produce more symptoms than other types of mediastinal neurogenic tumors, by direct local extension or compression of surrounding structures or catecholamine release. These tumors are very vascular and grossly tend to be unencapsulated, infiltrative lesions. Microscopically, packets of uniform cells, termed "Zellballen," are separated by highly vascular stromal trabeculae. The histologic appearance of functional and nonfunctional tumors is identical [11, 16].

Aortic body paragangliomas tend to occur in young adults, with an equal sex distribution. These tumors tend to extensively involve surrounding mediastinal structures. A high incidence of metastasis to lung, liver, or bone is noted. *Aorticosympathetic paragangliomas* are more common in the third to fifth decades of life, particularly among males. These neoplasms occur less frequently than aortic body paragangliomas and tend to be more localized. The incidence of metastases is low with such tumors. In both types of paraganglioma, the determination of benign or malignant subtype is dependent on findings of intrathoracic spread or unresectability, rather than or specific histologic criteria [16, 17].

10.4 Diagnosis

10.4.1 Symptoms

The majority of mediastinal neurogenic tumors are identified as asymptomatic lesions on a routine chest radiograph. The presence of symptoms in a patient with a mediastinal neurogenic tumor is typically associated with autonomic nervous or paraganglionic subtypes and/or malignancy. Symptoms may be divided into those associated with local tumor effects, typically related to pressure on or invasion into adjacent intrathoracic structures, and those due to systemic alterations induced by the release of biogenic amines or other substances (Table 10.2). All autonomic nervous and paraganglionic tumors have the potential for the production of biogenic amines. Patients with symptoms correlating with these substances may exhibit increased excretion of the products of catecholamine degradation (vanillylmandelic acid and homovanillic acid) in their urine [18].

Table 10.2. Symptoms of mediastinal neurogenic tumors

Local symptoms
Pain: local, neuritic, pleuritic
Cord compression: dumbbell tumor
Brachial plexus palsy
Horner's syndrome
Recurrent nerve palsy
Phrenic nerve palsy
Dyspnea
Dysphagia
Venous distention: cervicofacial, upper extremity
Upper extremity ischemia
Scoliosis
Chest wall deformity

Systemic symptoms
Hypertension
Cutaneous flushing
Diaphoresis
Diarrhea, abdominal distention
Weight loss
Failure to thrive

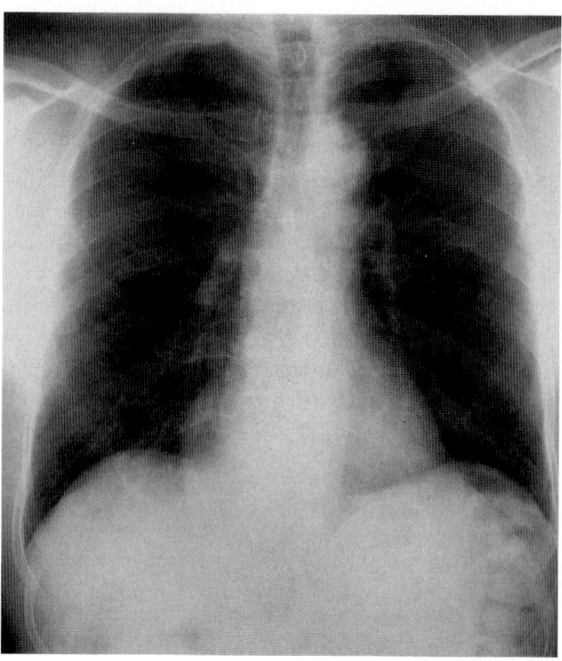

Fig. 10.1. Posteroanterior radiograph of the chest. A mass can be identified posterior to the right heart border, abutting the lower thoracic spine. The contour of the mass is ovoid, with a tapering cephalad margin. No sulcus sign is present. This lesion proved to be an autonomic nervous type of mediastinal neurogenic tumor (ganglioneuroma)

10.4.2 Radiographic Findings

Posteroanterior and lateral chest radiographs are the most common mode of identifying mediastinal neurogenic tumors. A rounded soft tissue density mass located in the posterior mediastinum has an 80% probability of being a mediastinal neurogenic tumor. The contour of the mass may correlate with the specific histologic classification of the neurogenic tumor. Nerve sheath tumors tend to be round with well-delineated borders. A sulcus effect is typically noted both above and below the tumor. Autonomic nervous tumors are ovoid and elongated, typically in a cephalad-caudad axis along the posterior sympathetic chain, with tapering or ill-defined borders (Fig. 10.1). A prominent sulcus is *not* seen, but other pleural changes, such as effusions or pleural nodules, may be noted [11].

Lobulation of the soft tissue mass is more common with tumors in NF patients, which have a higher incidence of malignancy, or with malignant autonomic nervous tumors. Homogeneous calcification may be seen about areas of cystic degeneration within nerve sheath tumors. A speckled calcification is occasionally seen with large ganglioneuromas [10, 11].

Mediastinal neurogenic tumors may cause multiple abnormalities in the bony thorax and vertebral column which may be identified on plain radiographs. Erosion of the inferior aspect of the head of the rib or splaying of the ribs may be seen with benign tumors. With excessive erosion, dis-location of the costovertebral junction may occur. Malignant neurogenic tumors, particularly autonomic nervous tumors, may exhibit frank rib invasion or destruction. The most common vertebral anomaly is enlargement of the intervertebral foramen, seen in 5% of patients. This finding suggests the possibility of intraspinal extension of the tumor and mandates further investigation. Thoracic dorsal scoliosis, away from the tumor, or developmental anomalies of the vertebral bodies may also be seen, more frequently with autonomic system tumors [5, 11].

Computed tomographic (CT) scanning of the chest has enhanced the sensitivity for the diagnosis of all mediastinal tumors. CT scans confirm the nature of the lesion, its contour characteristics, and its extent relative to surrounding structures. For malignant neurogenic tumors, potential sites of distant metastasis (e.g., pulmonary parenchyma, liver) may also be assessed. In addition, the CT scan allows limited assessment of the extent of rib and vertebral erosion or enlargement of the intervertebral foramen (Fig. 10.2). The final assessment of possible intraspinal extension of a posterior mediastinal tumor, however, is best obtained by magnetic resonance imaging (MRI) [8, 19].

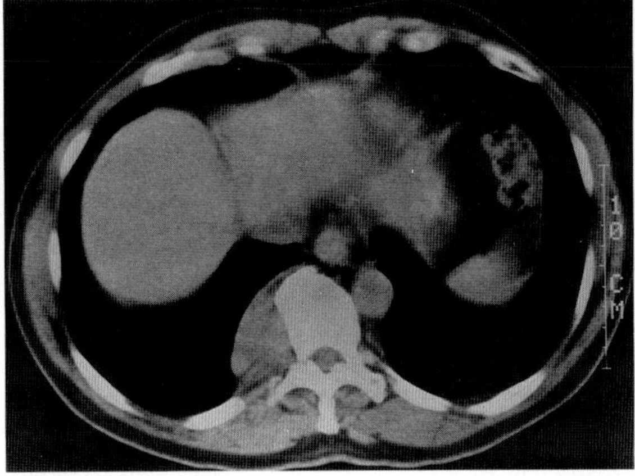

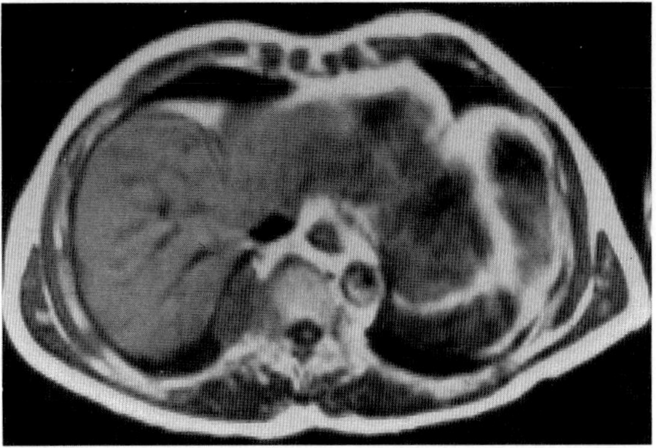

Fig. 10.2. CT scan of the chest. A mass arising in the right costovertebral sulcus can be identified. This mass proved to be a mediastinal neurogenic tumor. Erosion of the vertebral body is clearly evident. However, intraspinal extension cannot be definitively assessed

Fig. 10.3. MRI of the tumor demonstrated in Fig. 10.2. The extent of the tumor is much more clearly delineated in this study. Destruction of the vertebral pedicle and invasion through the intervertebral foramen are clearly seen. However, there is no evidence of direct cord compression

Magnetic resonance imaging may be superior to CT for evaluation of mediastinal neurogenic tumors because the coronal and sagittal as well as axial images enable precise identification of overall tumor extent. In the case of neurogenic tumors arising in the posterior mediastinum, of all histologic subtypes, the delineation of the neural structures of the spinal canal and the contrast discrimination between normal spinal cord and neoplastic tissue afforded by MRI make it the procedure of choice in evaluating the possibility of extension of such lesions into the spinal canal (Fig. 10.3). For the highly vascular paraganglionic tumors, MRI also provides information about the vascularity of the tumor (seen as a flow void on MRI studies) and allows easy distinction between the tumor and the great vessels when the site of origin is in the middle mediastinum [20].

Selective arteriography to identify the artery of Adamkiewicz supplying the anterior spinal artery has been recommended when intraspinal extension of a posterior mediastinal tumor is confirmed. This recommendation applies primarily to those tumors arising in the lower thorax, below the level of T6 [13].

The use of ^{131}I-metaiodobenzylguanidine scintigraphy has been shown to be very useful for the localization of paraganglionic tumors at both intrathoracic and extrathoracic sites. This technique has a false-positive rate of 0% and a false-negative rate of 10% for the diagnosis of paragangliomas, and may be used for primary delineation of paraganglionic tumors or for identification of possible multiple tumors in patients with known paragangliomas [21].

10.4.3 Needle Biopsy

A likely diagnosis of a mediastinal neurogenic tumor may be achieved from a judicious review of radiographic studies. However, a precise neoplastic classification can only be afforded by study of sufficient histologic material. Preoperative needle aspiration biopsy has been used for the diagnosis of mediastinal lesions in general. However, the use of this approach for mediastinal neurogenic tumors has been disappointing. A recent series reported insufficient tissue for evaluation in 50% of cases, although an 86% diagnostic accuracy was obtained when sufficient material was obtained [7]. Mediastinal neurogenic tumors of all types, including benign and malignant variants, will enlarge by definition and therefore have the potential for compression of adjacent vital intrathoracic structures. For this reason, the role of needle biopsy should be very limited, and surgical excision should be the primary modality for both diagnostic classification and therapy. In an analogous fashion, attempts at intraoperative determination of malignancy on the basis of histologic criteria may be extremely difficult, particularly for patients with NF. In such cases, en bloc excision of these tumors, within reasonable limits, is appropriate at the time of operative intervention upon identification of their neurogenic derivation, without further subclassification.

10.5 Treatment

Upon the presumptive diagnosis of a mediastinal neurogenic tumor, plans for preoperative assessment and surgical excision should be made. As noted previously, the majority of mediastinal neurogenic tumors, including both benign and malignant variants of all the histologic subtypes, are asymptomatic. The presence or absence of symptoms is not, therefore, a useful discriminator to determine the need for operative intervention. Even for benign lesions, should accurate confirmation be possible without formal surgical exposure, the potential for ongoing growth and involvement of adjacent structures limits the role of non-interventional therapy. Two notable exceptions to routine use of surgical excision for these tumors, however, are instances of extensive extrathoracic metastases (e.g., with neuroblastoma) and extensive infiltration of central vascular structures (e.g., with aortic body paraganglioma).

The majority of nerve sheath and autonomic system tumors, as well as the aorticosympathetic paragangliomas, are located in the posterior mediastinum. Upon determination of the absence of intraspinal extension, these lesions may be approached by a posterolateral thoracotomy. The intercostal incision is typically placed one or two interspaces above or below the lesion, to avoid injury to the neoplasm upon entering the thorax. An en bloc excision of the lesion and surrounding structures is performed. Autonomic nervous tumors tend to be more adherent than nerve sheath tumors and may also require limited resection of adherent tissues (e.g., wedge resection of lung) to obtain adequate margins of resection. Almost invariably, a nerve root must be sacrificed to complete excision of the neurogenic tumor. Division and ligation of adjacent intercostal vessels should be done judiciously, to prevent the possibility of retraction of the divided vessel into the spinal canal with subsequent hemorrhage and cord injury. For lesions arising within or adjacent to vital motor nerves (e.g., recurrent laryngeal nerve, brachial plexus), dissection with an operative microscope to preserve adjacent fibers may be necessary. The patient should be informed preoperatively of the potential for postoperative sensory or motor deficit due to these maneuvers. In addition, because of the variable course of resolution of compressive neuropathy, no assurance of the resolution of preoperative neurologic symptoms following excision of the tumor can be made.

Video-assisted thoracic surgery (VATS) has been used for identification and excision of mediastinal neurogenic tumors. Typically, the lesions have been well delineated by preoperative radiographic studies. The lesions have been visualized and mobilized using VATS and then removed via a minithoracotomy. VATS may be particularly advantageous for the visualization of tumors in the extreme cephalad portions of the posterior mediastinum [22]. However, for the majority of patients, a distinct advantage of VATS over open thoracotomy remains to be demonstrated. A VATS approach should be considered only for localized, presumably benign lesions by a surgeon with extensive advanced thoracoscopic experience.

Growth of neurogenic tumors medially from the posterior mediastinum through the intervertebral foramen into the spinal canal can result in a significant intracanal component of the tumor. The gross appearance of such a tumor, with a spherical portion at either end surrounding a narrowed region corresponding to the intervertebral foramen, has been described as a "dumbbell" shape [5]. The possibility of a dumbbell tumor should be entertained with *any* posterior mediastinal tumor. Dumbbell-shaped tumors are seen in 10% of mediastinal neurogenic tumors. Nerve sheath tumors account for 90% of neurogenic dumbbell tumors, although all histologic subtypes have been reported with this configuration [5, 23]. Symptoms of cord compression are seen in 60% of patients with these tumors; the remainder may be completely asymptomatic [24, 25]. Failure of preoperative identification of such a lesion may result in paraplegia following partial excision of only the intrathoracic component.

A single-stage, combined thoracic and neurosurgical approach is preferred for dumbbell tumors [5, 24]. The patient is placed in a lateral decubitus position and an L-shaped incision is created. The vertical portion of the incision is positioned over the spinous processes and extends 5 cm above and below the involved foramen. The transverse portion of the incision extends laterally to complete a standard thoracotomy incision. The skin and subcutaneous tissue within the confines of the incision are elevated and an intercostal incision is completed as previously described. After intrathoracic mobilization of the tumor up to the intervertebral foramen, the neurosurgical team performs a posterior laminectomy to gain access to the spinal canal. The tumor may be extradural or may require microsurgical dissection from the substance of the spinal cord. Upon completion of the excision, a vascularized flap of tissue is used to close the foramen and prevent intrathoracic leak of cerebrospinal fluid. An alternative approach is to place the patient prone and create a curvilinear paravertebral incision. This method may be especially useful for tumors with a large intraspinal component or those involving more than one intervertebral foramen [5, 19]. If resection of a dumbbell tumor is required in a pediatric patient, the procedure should be performed in conjuction with an orthopedic team to minimize the possibility of later kyphoscoliosis.

Median sternotomy is typically used for paraganglionic tumors of the middle mediastinum. Preoperative localization using MRI or scintigraphy is useful in determining the operative approach and/or resectability. On occasion, limited involvement of central vascular structures by these tumors may be resected using cardiopulmonary bypass techniques.

10.6 Prognosis

Complete excision of mediastinal neurogenic tumors conveys a very favorable prognosis. The survival following complete en bloc removal of benign lesions of any histologic type approaches 100%. The incidence of local recurrence of benign lesions removed in this fashion, by standard throacotomy, is negligible. Long-term follow-up for lesions treated by VATS is currently unavailable. When resection is not complete, and further resection is not possible, adjuvant radiation therapy may be of benefit. Radiation dosages of 20–40 Gy, corresponding to the amount of residual disease and the proximity of vital structures (e.g., spinal cord), are used. Despite residual tumor, prognosis remains acceptable with adjuvant radiotherapy. A 5-year survival of > 75% has been reported for benign nerve sheath and autonomic tumors treated in this fashion [5, 7].

Malignant neurogenic tumors that have been completely excised also have a favorable prognosis. Long-term survival following complete resection of malignant schwannoma has been reported [5]. For malignant autonomic nervous tumors 5-year survival figures of 88% and 80% have been reported for ganglioneuroblastoma and neuroblastoma, respectively [16, 26]. Completely excised malignant paragangliomas also have an excellent long-term prognosis. In many cases, however, complete excision of malignant mediastinal neurogenic tumors is not possible. Prognosis in these instances is generally poor. In the case of malignant schwannomas, despite aggressive adjuvant therapy, survival is less than 1 year. Residual ganglioneuroblastoma may be treated with adjuvant radiation therapy with an

outcome similar to that for incompletely excised benign neurogenic tumors. For incompletely excised or unresectable neuroblastomas, combination radiation and chemotherapy yields a long-term survival rate of 30%–40% [26]. Paragangliomas which are not completely excised are generally resistant to all forms of adjuvant therapy. All such patients are dead within 10 years of presentation [17].

References

1. Gould VE, Wiedemann B, Lee I, et al. (1987) Synaptophysin expression in neuroendocrine neoplasms as determined by immunocytochemistry. Am J Pathol 126: 243–240
2. Marangos PJ, Schmechel D (1980) The neurobiology of the brain enolase. In: Youdin MBH, Lovenberg W, Sharman DF, et al. (eds) Essays in neurochemistry and neuropharmacology, vol 4. Wiley, New York, pp 211–230
3. Enzinger FM, Weiss SW (1983) Benign tumors of peripheral nerves. In: Enzinger FJ, Weiss SW (eds) Soft tissue tumors. Mosby, St. Louis, pp 580–603
4. Ackerman LV, Taylor FH (1951) Neurogenous tumors within the thorax: a clinicopathologic evaluation of forty-eight cases. Cancer 4: 669–673
5. Akwari OE, Payne WS, Onofrio BM, et al. (1978) Dumbbell neurogenic tumors of the mediastinum. Mayo Clin Proc 53: 353–362
6. Adkins RB, Maples MD, Hainsworth JD (1984) Primary malignant mediastinal tumors (current review). Ann Thorac Surg 38: 648–655
7. Blegvad S, Lippert H, Simpler LB, Dybdahl H (1990) Mediastinal tumors: a report of 129 cases. Scan J Thorac Cardiovasc Surg 24: 39–44
8. Davis RD, Oldham HN, Sabiston DC (1987) Primary cysts and neoplasms of the mediastinum: recent changes in clinical presentation, methods of diagnosis, management and results. Ann Thorac Surg 44: 229–233
9. Carey LS, Ellis FH, Good CA, Woolner LB (1990) Neurogenic tumors of the mediastinum: a clinicopathologic study. AJR 84: 189–195
10. Davidson KG, Walbaum PR, McCormack RJM (1978) Intrathoracic neural tumours. Thorax 33: 359–364
11. Reed JC, Hallet KK, Feigin DS (1978) Neural tumors of the thorax: Subject review from the AFIP. Radiology 126: 9–18
12. Enzinger F (ed) (1969) Histologic typing of soft tissue tumours. WHO, Geneva, pp 23
13. Shields TW, Reynolds M (1988) Neurogenic tumors of the thorax. Surg Clin North Am 68: 645–651
14. Seeger RC, Siegel SE, Sidell N (1982) Neuroblastoma: Clinical perspectives, monoclonal antibodies and retinoic acid. Ann Intern Med 97: 873–877
15. Zajtchuk R, Bowen TE, Seyfer AE, Brott WH (1980) Intrathoracic ganglioneuroblastoma. J Thorac Cardiovasc Surg 80: 605–609
16. Adam A, Hochholzer L (1981) Ganglioneuroblastoma of the posterior mediastinum: a clinicopathologic review of 80 cases. Cancer 47: 373–381
17. Olson JL, Salyer WR (1978) Mediastinal paragangliomas (aortic body tumor): a report of four cases and a review of the literature. Cancer 41: 2105–2109

18. Hamilton JP, Koop CE (1965) Ganglioneuromas in children. Surg Gynecol Obstet 121:803–810
19. Ricci C, Rendina EA, Venuta F, et al. (1990) Diagnostic imaging and surgical treatment of dumbbell tumor of the mediastinum. Ann Thorac Surg 50:586–588
20. Tanaka F, Kitano M, Tatsumi A, et al. (1992) Paraganglioma of the posterior mediastinum: Value of magnetic resonance imaging 53:517–519
21. Shapiro B, Sisson J, Kalff V, et al. (1984) The location of middle mediastinal pheochromocytomas. J Thorac Cardiovasc Surg 87:814–821
22. Coosemans W, Lerut TE, Van Raemdonck DEM (1993) Thoracoscopic surgery: the Belgian experience. Ann Thorac Surg 56:721–730
23. Heuer GJ (1929) The so-called hour-glass tumors of the spine. Arch Surg 18:935–942
24. Grillo HC, Ojemann RG, Scannnell JG, Zervas NT (1983) Combined approach to "dumbbell" intrathoracic and intraspinal neurogenic tumors. Ann Thorac Surg 36:402–407
25. Wain JC (1992) Neurogenic tumors of the mediastinum In: Benfield JR (ed) Mediastinal tumors – chest surgery clinics of North America. Saunders, Philadelphia, pp 121–136
26. McGuire WA, Simmons D, Grosfeld JL, et al. (1985) Stage II neuroblastoma: does adjuvant irradiation contribute to cure? Med Pediatr Oncol 13:117–125

11 Cardiac Neoplasms

CHARLES R. THOMAS, JR., BRENT DE VRIES, JACOB D. BITRAN, and THOMAS W. GRIFFIN

CONTENTS

11.1 Introduction

Cardiac tumors are rare and the majority are benign [1]. In the era prior to echocardiography and cardiac

CHARLES R. THOMAS, JR., M.D., Fellow, Department of Radiation Oncology, University of Washington School of Medicine, 1959 NE Pacific Street, Seattle, WA 98195, USA
BRENT DE VRIES, D.O., Fellow, Division of Cardiology, Department of Medicine, Lutheran General Hospital, Park Ridge, IL 60068-1129, USA
JACOB D. BITRAN, M.D., Clinical Professor of Medicine, Division of Hematology/Oncology, Department of Medicine, Lutheran General Hospital, Park Ridge, IL 60068-1129, USA
THOMAS W. GRIFFIN, M.D., Professor and Chairman, Department of Radiation Oncology, University of Washington School of Medicine, 1959 NE Pacific Street, Seattle, WA 98195, USA

catheterization, the diagnosis of a cardiac tumor was made only at autopsy. With the advances in imaging modalities and improvements in surgical techniques, patients with these neoplasms may be potentially treatable. The clinician must have a high index of suspicion if a diagnosis of a cardiac neoplasm is to be made since the related clinical symptom complex usually mimics other nonneoplastic cardiac disease [2]. As a consequence, primary cardiac neoplasms have been referred to as the "great imitators" of the cardiovascular system [3].

Cardiac neoplasms can be subdivided into primary and metastatic tumors of the heart. Metastatic tumors are found 20–30 times more frequently than primary cardiac tumors. Of the primary tumors of the heart, 75% are benign, with myxomas accounting for 50%–60% of all primary cardiac tumors [1].

11.2 Benign Cardiac Tumors

11.2.1 Overview

There are a variety of nonspecific clinical findings associated with cardiac tumors. Generalized weakness, weight loss, malaise, easy fatigability, and dyspnea are common symptoms. Focal symptoms and signs can be grouped according to the anatomic location of cardiac involvement.

1. *Pericardial involvement.* Tumor spread to this area can result in pericarditis or pericardial effusion manifested by chest pain, palpitations, and dyspnea [2]. Other findings include a pericardial friction rub and increased jugular venous pulsation. Electrocardiography and chest radiography may suggest cardiomegaly.

2. *Myocardial involvement.* Myocardial involvement is characterized by a wide variety of symptoms. These patients frequently have supraventricular and ventricular tachyarrhythmias [2]. With invasion of the ventricular wall these patients may complain of chest pain. There may be a suggestion of myocardial

infarction on electrocardiography. Conduction abnormalities and atrioventricular block, when present, may present with sudden death.

3. *Endocardial involvement.* Left atrial tumors may prolapse into the mitral valve orifice, causing outflow obstruction and mitral regurgitation, mimicking mitral valve disease – especially mitral stenosis.

11.2.2 Myxomas

Myxomas are the most common of all cardiac tumors [4, 5]. Most patients are between 30 and 60 years of age and 70% are women. Seventy-five percent of the myxomas occur in the left atrium, whereas only 25% are found in the right atrium. Most myxomas are solitary tumors; however, multiple tumors, in either a single chamber or a combination of chambers, also may occur.

Myxomas are pedunculated with a fibrovascular stalk. They typically have a gelatinous consistency and are lobulated with an average size that ranges between 4 and 8 cm [2].

Physical examination may be consistent with left ventricular failure. Auscultation may reveal a "tumor plop" which is caused by the tumor striking the endocardial wall or the abrupt stop of the tumor. Right-sided lesions may elicit symptoms of right heart failure such as fatigue, peripheral edema, ascites, hepatomegaly, and an increase in jugular venous pulsation which is the result of interference with the tricuspid valve. Pulmonary embolus or pulmonary hypertension is another complication of right-sided tumors and simulates thomboembolic events.

Surgical resection is the treatment of choice for myxomas [2]. Tumor fragments may dislodge during the operation, which can result in peripheral embolization and seeding of metastases. Locally recurrent and invasive myxomas as well as distant metastases from myxomas have been reported. Although usually benign, myxomas may demonstrate malignant potential.

11.2.2.1 Familial Cardiac Myxomas

A subset of patients with myxomas has also been identified [6]. These cases may be familial and transmitted in an autosomal dominant type of pattern. Familial cardiac myxomas are associated with pigmented skin lesions and have been described in

association with extracardiac endocrine neoplasms [2]. Generally, patients with "syndrome" myxomas are younger and more likely to have multiple myxomas involving cardiac chambers other than the left atrium. They also have a higher incidence of recurrent myxomas postoperatively.

Certain aspects of the "myxoma syndrome" have been referred to as the NAME syndrome (*n*evi, *a*trial myxoma, *m*yxoid neurofibroma, and blue nevi) and the LAMB syndrome (*l*entigines, *a*trial *m*yxoma, and *b*lue nevi) [7–9]. Associated with the familial or complex myxomas are skin lesions (ephelides, blue nevi, or lentigines), skin myxomas, myxoid mammary fibroadenosis, Cushing's syndrome, pituitary adenomas, testicular thyroid, and uterine tumors [10]. Hematologic abnormalities include hemolytic anemia and thrombocytopenia.

The age of patients with the myxoma syndrome is 22–30 years. Most patients with the myxoma syndrome have first-degree relatives with one or more elements of the syndrome complex. Therefore, routine echocardiographic screening of first-degree relatives is appropriate. A single myxoma occurs in about one-third of these patients and following surgical resection the recurrence rate is 20%.

11.2.3 Rhabdomyoma

Rhabdomyoma is the second most common benign cardiac tumor and is the most common cardiac tumor of childhood [2]. Rhabdomyomas are strongly associated with tuberous sclerosis (a familial syndrome characterized by hamartomas, epilepsy, mental deficiency, and adenoma sebaceum). They are usually multiple and involve the ventricles more often than the atria. The presentation may be as an intramural lesion or an intracavitary mass. A history of heart failure or tachyarrhythmias is not uncommon. The majority of patients diagnosed during infancy do not survive for more than a year. Surgical resection of rhabdomyomas localized to the ventricle has yielded good results [2].

11.2.4 Fibroma

Fibromas of the heart are connective tissue tumors that occur predominantly in children. The majority occur before the age of 10 years, with males and females being affected equally. Fibromas are usually located in the ventricular myocardium. Clinical manifestations include chest pain, syncope, and sudden death. Arrhythmias are found in at least one-third of patients, with sudden death being reported secondary to ventricular tachyarrhythmias [2]. Cardiac calcification may be present on chest radiograph. The Gorlin syndrome, whose features are multiple nevoid basal cell carcinomas, cysts of the jaw, and skeletal abnormalities, may also be associated with fibromas or fibrous histiocytomas [11].

These tumors are circumscribed but not encapsulated. As with the other benign tumors of the heart, surgical resection is desirable and is associated with good long-term survival. Orthotopic cardiac transplantation has been used occasionally to treat patients with unresectable disease [12].

11.2.5 Lipoma

Lipomas may occur throughout the heart, including the pericardium. They occur at all ages with equal frequency in males and females. Intramyocardial tumors are encapsulated and usually small. Intrapericardial tumors may be large and can cause pericardial effusion [2]. Lipomas may also present as asymptomatic cardiomegaly or mediastinal enlargement. Surgical resection has yielded good long-term results.

Lipomatous hypertrophy of the interatrial system is a nonencapsulated hyperplasia of mature adipose tissue which results in the adipose tissue protruding into the right atrium [2]. It usually occurs in obese, elderly, or female patients. Supraventricular arrhythmia and conduction disturbances are common consequences.

11.2.6 Hemangioma

Hemangiomas are rare cardiac tumors. They occur mainly in adults and are usually found incidentally at autopsy [2]. Hemangiomas may be located in all parts of the heart but usually are intramural. They may present as diffuse proliferations rather than distinct tumors and consequently total excision is often not feasible.

11.2.7 Teratomas

Teratomas contain elements derived from all three germ cell layers. Most commonly they occur in the anterior mediastinum. When they do develop in the heart, the right-sided chambers and the interatrial or interventricular septum are the most common locations. These tumors are well encapsulated but have malignant potential.

11.2.8 Papillary Fibroelastoma

Papillary fibroelastomas are rare and usually arise from cardiac valves of occasionally the ventricular endocardium [2]. Most commonly they are incidental findings at surgery or at autopsy. Complications of this tumor include valvular dysfunction, sudden death, and embolic events. Embolic material may arise from either tumor fragments or thrombi that form around the tumor. Surgical excision is required to prevent these complications.

11.2.9 Endocrine Tumors

Paragangliomas (pheochromocytomas, chemodectomas) are very rare tumors of the pericardium. They may occur in epicardium of the left-sided chambers and are thought to arise from sympathetic fibers to the heart or ectopic chromaffin cells. These tumors may secrete catecholamines and can be associated with the signs and symptoms of pheochromocytoma.

11.3 Primary Malignant Cardiac Tumors

11.3.1 Overview

Approximately one-fourth of all cardiac tumors are malignant. Most primary malignant cardiac (PMC) neoplasms are sarcomas [13]. These tumors are rapidly progressive. Death may occur within a few weeks after the onset of symptoms. About 80% of patients have systemic metastases at the time of diagnosis. Rapid infiltration through the myocardium is particularly characteristic of mesothelioma. The majority of patients will have clinical evidence of right heart failure since most PMC tumors originate from the right side of the heart. Chest pain, fever, and, if obstruction of the superior vena cava occurs, swelling of the face and extremities are present. If there is extension into the pericardial space, tamponade may become rapidly evident. In general, the prognosis is poor, with few long-term survivors reported [2, 13].

11.3.2 Angiosarcoma

Angiosarcomas are the most common PMC tumor [13, 14]. They are more common in males and usually present in the fourth to fifth decade of life [15]. The right atrium is the most common cardiac site of involvement [13, 16]. As the tumor grows within the atrial wall, a large intracavitary projection may be appreciated [13]. Venae cavae or tricuspid valve outflow tract compromise may also develop.

Pathologic examination reveals a tumor with characteristic vascular channel formation. Angiosarcomas initially involve the epicardial layer, followed by transmural infiltration through the myocardium and eventually extending into the endocardium [17]. Extension into the subepicardial fat may occur with the Kaposi's sarcoma subtype [18].

On examination, most patients present with evidence of right-sided heart failure and seldom are pathologic murmurs noted [13]. Chest radiography and echocardiography will show evidence of cardiomegaly and pericardial effusion, along with a right atrial mass [16].

The rapid course of this tumor often results in the diagnosis being established postmortem [16, 19]. Most angiosarcomas of the heart eventually spread of the lungs, the mediastinal and parietal pleurae, mediastinal lymph nodes, and liver, in descending order of frequency [13, 17, 20]. The cause of death is usually local extension outward into the pericardial sac, as evidenced by gross tumor or an organized hemorrhage [17].

A complete surgical resection is seldom possible, necessitating the use of postoperative chemotherapy and radiation [13, 20, 21]. Palliative procedures often yield immediate symptomatic relief. Reconstruction of the cardiac chambers and valve replacement are often required [22]. Few patients live beyond 6 months from the time of surgery [13, 16].

11.3.3 Rhabdomyosarcoma

Rhabdomyosarcomas are the second most frequent PMC tumor, usually occurring between the third and fifth decades [1, 13]. This tumor is found in all four cardiac chambers with equal frequency. The sex ratio is also equal [13]. Intracavitary lesions are likely to spread directly into adjacent valves, most commonly the pulmonic or mitral. Up to half will have pericardial involvement. Most patients will present with signs of heart failure. As with angiosarcomas, surgical resection is rarely curative, since

most of these tumors have spread by the time a tissue diagnosis has been obtained [13, 23, 24]. When possible postoperative chemotherapy and radiation should be administered.

11.3.4 Fibrosarcoma

Fibrosarcomas are next in frequency and are most common during the second and third decades [25]. There is a slight predilection for females and for a left-sided location, specifically along the posterior wall and/or septum of the left atrium [13, 25, 26]. The mitral valve is frequently involved directly, with the left ventricular outflow tract eventually becoming compromised [13]. An association between prior mitral valve replacement and the development of fibrosarcoma has been proposed, though causation has been difficult to prove [27]. Most patients present in left heart failure [13, 28]. Once again, overall survival is dismal, although 2 + year survivors have been reported [29, 30]. Surgical resection, followed by careful administration of anthracycline-based adjuvant chemotherapy and localized radiation, should be attempted [13, 26].

11.3.5 Lymphoma

Because of the paucity of lymphoid tissue in the heart it is extremely difficult to prove that any lymphomatous involvement does not originate from an extracardiac site. Slightly more than a quarter of extracardiac lymphomas will eventually metastasize to the heart. If a lymphoma originates as a true PMC tumor, it is likely to metastasize early on [13]. Most are of a high grade, non-Hodgkin's B-cell variety [31, 32]. When the lymphoma is diagnosed, treatment involves combination chemotherapy, which is potentially curative [33]. Unfortunately, the inability to diagnose these tumors antemortem has limited the use of such useful therapy.

11.3.6 Mesothelioma

The pericardium is the most common site of cardiac involvement by mesothelioma. No clear association with asbestos has been demonstrated [13]. Both the visceral and the parietal pericardium is usually involved, with distant metastasis a less likely sequela. Patients usually present with characteristic pleuritic chest discomfort, dyspnea, and an overall clinical picture supportive of constrictive pericarditis. An echocardiogram will often show evidence of impairment to diastolic filling [13]. A pericardiocentesis yields the diagnosis. Successful stripping of the pericardium is uncommon and there are no routinely active chemotherapeutic agents. Mesothelioma does not respond to radiotherapy. As a result, long-term prognosis is often completely dependent on medical management of diastolic dysfunction.

Mesothelioma of the atrioventricular node is capable of causing sudden death via complete heart block or ventricular fibrillation. This occurs most frequently in adult females. The PMC tumor is generally less than 15 mm in diameter. Mesotheliomas usually present during the first or second decade, and frequently are noted at the time of puberty or during pregnancy. Electronic pacing may be required to prevent sudden death [34].

11.4 Treatment of Primary Malignant Cardiac Tumors

11.4.1 Radiotherapy

Clear margins are rarely obtained from surgical resection. When margins are obtained, there may be only a few millimeters separating normal cardiac tissue from the tumor edge. In most instances, there has been occult spread already. As a result, multimodal therapy, involving adjuvant external beam radiotherapy, is advocated [13, 35].

A daily dose of 1.8 Gy in 28 fractions, up to a total dose of 50.4 Gy, should be given adjuvantly for sarcoma subtypes [16, 30, 35]. A 10-Gy boost can sometimes be given to very limited areas of the heart. For rare lymphomatous PMC tumors, doses of 15–20 Gy may be more appropriate, since effective chemotherapy may decrease the need for higher radiotherapy doses. The treatment volume must include the whole pericardium with a 2-cm margin. The middle and lower mediastinum should be included in the treatment volume in order to address the mediastinal lymph node basin [35].

While anthracyclines, such as doxorubicin, have shown efficacy for many sarcomas, the optimal sequencing with radiation is unclear.

11.4.2 Chemotherapy

Dacarbazine and doxorubicin are the two most active chemotherapeutic agents for sarcomas. Ifosfamide, an alkylating agent analog of cyclophosphamide, has demonstrated activity in previously treated extracardiac sarcomas and is often used as a front-line agent at some centers. Cisplatin may also have activity.

The few patients with PMC tumors who have been healthy enough to receive combination chemotherapy have responded to treatment [13]. Those who have lived longest had previously undergone a complete surgical resection. Radiotherapy is often necessary if long-term survival is to be even remotely expected. Unfortunately, unlike germ cell tumors or lymphomas, chemotherapy alone will not result in definitive killing of the tumor clone. Multiple drug resistance quickly develops as the disease progresses.

11.4.3 Surgery

Surgical resection is the mainstay of therapy for PMC tumors. A myriad of surgical interventions have been utilized [13]. The type of operation depends on the location and extent of disease. Cardiopulmonary bypass and arrest with cardioplegia allows for the direct visualization and necessary palpation of the tumor in a clearer operative field. It is critical that the extent of the tumor's attachment to underlying tissue be appreciated prior to resection. If clear margins cannot be obtained due to the proximity of other vital structures, a debulking procedure should be attempted in order to palliate the presenting symptoms. Orthotopic transplantation and autotransplantation have also been utilized [12, 36, 37].

11.5 Prognostic Factors for Primary Malignant Cardiac Tumors

While most PMC tumors are uniformly fatal, there are some features that may predict a more favorable outcome [13, 38]:

1. Location to one cardiac chamber without involvement of the neighboring valve
2. Presence of a low mitotic index on histologic examination
3. Lack of tumor necrosis
4. Tumors located in the left heart
5. Good performance status postoperatively which allows radiation and chemotherapy to be given.

11.6 Metastatic Tumors of the Heart and Pericardium

Cardiac metastases are more common than primary cardiac tumors [13,15]. These metastatic tumors occur with almost all types of malignancies. Metastatic involvement has been found in up to one-fifth of patients at autopsy who have lung, esophageal, or breast cancer primaries. Malignant melanoma involves the myocardium in more than 50% of cases. Involvement from hematologic malignancies has been reported to be less common.

Hematogenous embolic dissemination is the main route of metastasis to the heart. Lymphatic spread and direct invasion by tumor occur less often. Secondary involvement of the heart is a common autopsy finding in patients with widespread metastasis, when looked for. Less than one-third of patients exhibit cardiac symptoms, and clinical findings associated with metastatic cardiac lesions include pericardial effusion, cardiomegaly, ventricular failure, and arrhythmias. A large pericardial effusion may evolve into cardiac tamponade.

Arrhythmias are common signs of myocardial involvement. As more myocardium becomes infiltrated with tumor, heart failure develops. Some metastatic lesions may be intracavitary and direct valvular involvement with obstruction can occur. Acute myocardial infarction may occur by either external tumor compression of a coronary artery or coronary occlusion due to tumor embolization. Additionally, infarction may occur from coronary fibrosis or accelerated atherosclerosis in the patient who has received radiation to the mediastinum.

11.7 Conclusion

Most tumors involving chambers and valvular apparatus of the heart are metastatic deposits from an extracardiac site. While most of the lesions are subclinical, some may result in a clinical presentation that mimics cerebrovascular disease or congestive heart failure. Lesions involving the pericardium usually produce pleuritic chest discomfort, indicative of a pericardial effusion.

Primary tumors of the heart and pericardium are rare. Most lesions are benign, with left atrium myxomas being most common. Of the malignant tumors, angiosarcoma and mesothelioma are most common, being located in the right atrium and pericardium, respectively.

A high degree of clinical suspicion is required in order to arrive at an antemortem diagnosis. The availability of two-dimensional echocardiography and magnetic resonance imaging, along with cardiac catheterization, has allowed cardiac tumors to be better characterized over the past decade.

Surgical resection is the mainstay of treatment for both benign and malignant lesions. Chemotherapy and radiation therapy should be administered postoperatively in most good performance status patients with primary malignant cardiac tumors.

References

1. McAllister HA, Fenoglio JJ (1978) Tumors of the cardiovascular system. In: Atlas of tumor pathology, 2nd series, fascicle 15. Armed Forces Institute of Pathology, Washington
2. Hall RJ, Cooley DA, McAllister JA Jr, Frazier OH (1994) Neoplastic heart disease. In: Schlant RC, Alexander RW, O'Rourke RA, Roberts R, Sonnenblick EH (eds) The heart, arteries, and veins, 8th edn. McGraw-Hill, New York, pp 2007–2029
3. Goodwin JF (1968) The spectrum of cardiac tumors. Am J Cardiol 21: 307–314
4. Goldman AP, Kotler MN, Parry WR (1986) Atrial tumors. In: Kapoor AS (ed) Cancer and the heart. Springer, New York Berlin Heidelberg, pp 101–109
5. Harvey WP (1968) Clinical aspects of cardiac tumors. Am J Cardiol 21: 328
6. Powers JC, Falkoff M, Heinle RA, et al. (1979) Familial cardiac myxoma: emphasis on unusual clinical manifestations. J Thorac Cardiovasc Surg 77: 782–788
7. Atherton DJ, Pitcher DW, Wells RS, MacDonald DM (1980) A syndrome of various cutaneous pigmented lesions, myxoid neurofibromata and atrial myxoma: the NAME syndrome. Br J Dermatol 103: 421–429
8. Koopman RJJ, Happle R (1991) Autosomal dominant transmission of the NAME syndrome (nevi, atrial myxoma, mucinosis of the skin and endocrine overactivity). Hum Genet 86: 300–304
9. Rhodes AR, Silverman RA, Harris TJ, Perez-Atayde AR (1984) Mucocutaneous lentigines, cardiomucocutaneous myxomas, and multiple blue nevi: the LAMB syndrome. J Am Acad Dermatol 10: 72–82
10. Ichiba Y, Nishizaki Y, Tanizaki M (1992) Cushing's syndrome due to primary pigmented nodular adrenocortical disease with cardiac myxomas and mucocutaneous lentigines. Acta Paediatr 81: 91–92
11. Jones KL, Wolf PL, Jensen P, Dittrich H, Benirschke K, Bloor C (1986) The Gorlin syndrome: a genetically determined disorder associated with cardiac tumor. Am Heart J 111: 1013
12. Jamieson SW, Gaudiani BA, Reitz GA, et al. (1981) Operative treatment of an unresectable tumor of the left ventricle. J Thorac Cardiovasc Surg 81: 797–799
13. Thomas CR Jr, Johnson GW Jr, Stoddard MF, Clifford S (1992) Primary malignant cardiac tumors: update 1992. Med Pediatr Oncol 20: 519–531
14. Silverman N (1980) Primary cardiac tumors. Ann Surg 191: 127–138

15. Wilding G, Green H, Longo D, Urba W (1988) Tumors of the heart and pericardium. Cancer Treat Rev 25: 165–181
16. Herrmann MA, Shankerman RA, Edwards WD, Shub C, Schaff HV (1992) Primary cardiac angiosarcoma: a clinico-pathologic study of six cases. J Thorac Cardiovasc Surg 103: 655–664
17. Glancey DL, Morales JB, Roberts WC (1968) Angiosarcoma of the heart. Am J Cardiol 21: 413
18. Silver MA, Macher AM, Reichert CM, Levens DL, Parillo JE, Longo DL, et al. (1984) Cardiac involvement by Kaposi's sarcoma in acquired immune deficiency syndrome (AIDS). Am J Cardiol 53: 983–985
19. Klima U, Wimmer-Greinecker G, Harringer W, Mair R, Grob C, Brucke P (1993) Cardiac angiosarcoma – a diagnostic dilemma. Cardiovasc Surg 1: 674–676
20. Janigan DT, Husain A, Robinson NA (1986) Cardiac angiosarcomas: a review and a case report. Cancer 57: 852–859
21. Miralles A, Bracamonte L, Soncul H, del Castillo RD, Akhtar R, Bors V, et al. (1991) Cardiac tumors: clinical experience and surgical results in 74 patients. Ann Thorac Surg 52: 886–895
22. Dein JR, Frist WH, Stinson EB, et al. (1987) Primary cardiac neoplasms: early and late results of surgical treatment in 42 patients. J Thorac Cardiovasc Surg 93: 502–511
23. Chaudron JMS, Saint-Remy J-M, Schmitz A, Labacq EG (1977) Right atrium rhabdomyosarcoma. Acta Cardiol 32: 75–81
24. Matloff JM, Bass H, Dalen JE (1971) Rhabdomyosarcoma of the left atrium. Physiologic responses to surgical therapy. J Thorac Cardiovasc Surg 61: 451–455
25. Laya MB, Mailliard JA, Bewtra C, Levin HS (1987) Malignant fibrous histiocytoma of the heart: a case report and review of the literature. Cancer 59: 1026–1031
26. Wahba A, Liebold A, Birnbaum DE (1993) Recurrent malignant fibrous histiocytoma of the left atrium in a 27-year-old male. Eur J Cardiothorac Surg 7: 387–389
27. Holtzman E, Schiby G, Segal P, Priel I (1986) Malignant fibrous histiocytoma complicating mitral valve replacement. J Am Coll Cardiol 7: 956–960
28. Knobel B, Rosman P, Kishon Y, Husar M (1992) Intracardiac primary fibrosarcoma. Case report and literature review. Thorac Cardiovasc Surg 40: 227–230
29. Ecksteine R, Gossner W, Rienmuller R (1984) Primary malignant fibrous histiocytoma of the left atrium: surgical and chemotherapeutic management. Br Heart J 52: 354–357
30. Stevens CW, Sears-Rogan P, Bitterman P, Torrisi J (1992) Treatment of malignant fibrous histiocytoma of the heart. Cancer 69: 956–961
31. Balasubramanyam A, Waxman M, Kazal HL, Lee MH (1986) Malignant lymphoma of the heart in acquired immune deficiency syndrome. Chest 90: 243–246
32. Scully RE, Mark EJ, McNeely BV (1985) Case records of the Massachusetts General Hospital: case 4-1985. N Engl J Med 312: 226–237
33. Zaharia L, Gill PS (1991) Primary cardiac lymphoma. Am J Clin Oncol 14: 142–145
34. James TN, Galakhov I (1977) De subitaneis mortibus. XXVI. Fatal electrical instability of the heart associated with benign congenital polycystic tumor of the atrioventricular node. Circulation 6: 667–678
35. Emami B, Antoniades J (1992) Heart and blood vessels. In: Perez CA, Brady LW (eds), Principles and practice of radiation oncology, 2nd edn. Lippincott, Philadelphia, pp 871–876
36. Cooley DA, Peardon MJ, Frazier OH, et al. (1985) Human cardiac transplantation and autotransplantation: application in a patient with a large cardiac pheochromocytoma. Texas Heart Inst J 12: 171–176
37. Murphy MC, Sweeney MS, Putnam JB Jr, et al. (1990) Surgical treatment of cardiac tumors: a 25-year experience. Ann Thorac Surg 49: 612–618
38. Burke AP, Cowan D, Virmani R (1992) Primary sarcomas of the heart. Cancer 69: 387–395

12 Tracheal Tumors

DOUGLAS E. WOOD

CONTENTS

12.1 Introduction

Tumors of the trachea are extremely uncommon, with an estimated 2.6 new cases per million each year [1], translating to an estimated 600–700 cases each year in the United States. Tracheal tumors represent only 0.2% of all malignancies of the respiratory tract [2], with tumors of the larynx, bronchi, and lung occurring 75, 100, and 180 times more frequently, respectively [3, 4]. Though there are many case reports of tracheal tumors in both the otolaryngology and thoracic surgery literature, there are few large series, most notably those by ESCHAPASSE [5], GRILLO [6, 7], GRILLO and MATHISEN [8], PEARSON et al. [9], PERELMAN and KOROLEVA [10, 11], and XU et al. [12]. Due to the rarity of these tumors, as well as the diversity of pathology, even the larger series are unable to provide definitive data about the long-range results of treatment. These studies have accrued patients over many years, during which there have been many improvements in both surgical technique and radiation therapy.

Tracheal tumors are more common in men than in women [13]. However, when divided by pathologic diagnosis, squamous cell carcinoma occurs predominantly in men, while adenoid cystic carcinoma and miscellaneous tumors show an even distribution between the sexes [8]. Squamous cell carcinoma is primarily a disease of smokers with a peak incidence in the sixth and seventh decades. Adenoid cystic tumors show a fairly even age distribution from the third to the seventh decade and the variety of other tumors can present throughout life, including childhood and adolescence [8].

12.2 Assessment

The symptoms and signs of tracheal tumors are insidious in onset and are usually misdiagnosed for several months before a diagnosis is made. Symptoms consist of dyspnea, hemoptysis, cough, wheezing, dysphagia, stridor, hoarseness, or pneumonia [14]. Though the physical examination may be normal, patients may have a protracted sternal murmur, stridor, wheezing, and a weak or hoarse voice from diminished air flow across the vocal cords or involvement of the recurrent laryngeal nerve [11, 13]. Patients are often treated with increasingly aggressive regimens for refractory adult-onset asthma leading to progression of disease and presentation with critical airway obstruction [3, 12–14]. It is very important for the clinician to have a high index of suspicion when faced with these symptoms, or refractory "asthma," to make the correct diagnosis.

Patients suspected of having a tracheal neoplasm should undergo a routine PA and lateral chest x-ray, which in some cases can confirm the diagnosis of an intraluminal mass (Fig. 12.1). An overpenetrated high kV view of the trachea, AP, lateral, and oblique tomograms, and fluoroscopy can further define the presence of a tumor as well as its location, length, and relation to neighboring structures [14]. Patients with symptoms of dysphagia should undergo a barium esophagogram to define esophageal involvement. Computed tomography is very important in the evaluation of tracheal masses and is most useful to determine the extraluminal extent of the tumor and the presence of enlarged lymph nodes (Fig. 12.2). However, it is also useful in adding information regarding the extent and

DOUGLAS E. WOOD, M.D., Head, Section of General Thoracic Surgery, and Assistant Professor, Division of Cardiothoracic Surgery, SA-25, University of Washington, Seattle, WA 98195, USA

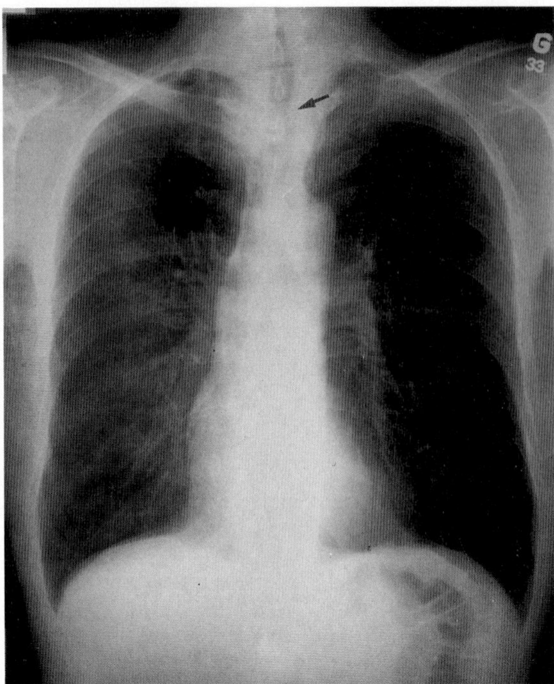

Fig. 12.1. PA chest radiograph demonstrates a midtracheal soft tissue mass (*arrow*) in a 57-year-old man with hemoptysis. Pathology showed a squamous cell carcinoma, which was completely resected and followed by adjuvant radiation therapy

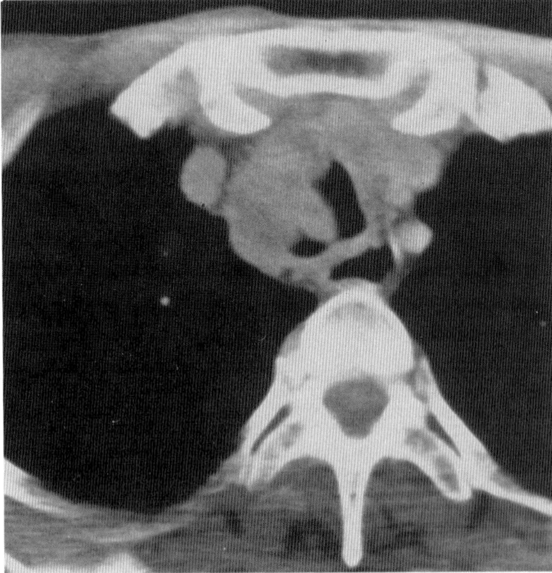

Fig. 12.2. Chest CT of the upper mediastinum demonstrates nearly circumferential involvement of the trachea by an adenoid cystic carcinoma. Though there is extension of tumor into the mediastinum, there is no evidence of invasion into other structures precluding surgical resection

location of the intraluminal tumor though the conventional tomograms are usually more sensitive and are especially important for surgical planning due to the good definition of longitudinal extent of disease and relationship to important anatomic landmarks. Magnetic resonance imaging seldom adds additional information though it is sometimes helpful in assessing the extent of the disease due to the multiplanar imaging capabilities.

Bronchoscopy is essential in the diagnosis and management of tracheal tumors. It is important for detection, histologic diagnosis, surgical planning, relief of acute obstruction, and palliation. When a tracheal tumor is suspected, but not confirmed by radiologic studies, the patient should undergo a diagnostic bronchoscopy to confirm or exclude the presence of an endobronchial mass. However, most tracheal surgeons feel that if a radiologically well-defined tumor appears resectable, bronchoscopy should be delayed until the time of definitive therapy to avoid precipitating acute airway obstruction [13, 15–17]. Others prefer to plan surgery with a histologic diagnosis and perform bronchoscopy as a separate preliminary procedure [11]. It is a common misconception that biopsy of tracheal tumors is hazardous and may result in life-threatening hemorrhage [11, 13, 17]. However, when vascular tumors such as hemangiomas, arteriovenous malformations, and some carcinoids are avoided, massive bleeding is unusual [18]. When bleeding does occur, it can almost always be managed through the rigid bronchoscope, which can be used to maintain the airway, suction aspirated blood, and tamponade or laser bleeding points. In this setting, bronchoscopy should be performed in the operating room with the capability of controlling the airway with a rigid bronchoscope or, if necessary, converting to a definitive open procedure.

Rigid bronchoscopy should be performed before a planned surgical resection to achieve the most accurate assessment of the tumor and its location and extent. Careful measurements of the length of involved trachea as well as the distance from important landmarks, such as the cricoid and the carina, are critical to determining operability and the optimal operative approach. There is no absolute guide to the maximum length of trachea that can be resected. In ideal conditions it may be possible to resect up to one-half of the trachea and achieve a primary reconstruction. Due to the restriction of the aortic arch on proximal mobilization of the left mainstem bronchus, usually only 4 cm can be resected at the carina with plans for a carinal reconstruction. Factors such as advanced age, kyphosis, short neck, poor neck mobility, and previous surgery or radiation may adversely affect the length of trachea that may be removed and primarily reconstructed. Since there is no prosthetic substitute for the trachea, these factors must be weighed carefully by the surgeon before undertaking attempts at surgical resection.

Patients with tracheal tumors may present with critical airway narrowing, stridor, respiratory distress, and obstructive pneumonia. Many of these tumors will be resectable with modern bronchoplastic techniques but require urgent or emergent relief of airway obstruction. This will allow time for further workup, stabilization, weaning from steroids, and clearing of pneumonia before undergoing surgical resection [18]. In these cases the rigid bronchoscope and biopsy forceps can be used to "core-out" the tumor with successful improvement in the airway in nearly all patients with tumor limited to the trachea or mainstem bronchi [18]. When the tumor extends distally into lobar and segmental bronchi, the results are much less predictable. Though the CO_2 or Nd:YAG laser can be a useful adjunct to this procedure, it seldom improves on the results obtainable by mechanical coring-out of tumor alone [18]. In those cases where the length of disease or invasion of surrounding structures precludes tracheal resection and reconstruction, these same bronchoscopic techniques for relief of obstruction, combined with stents and T-tubes, can provide excellent palliation (see below).

In cases that may involve the esophagus, preoperative esophagoscopy is essential to exclude transmural esophageal invasion. Occasionally mediastinoscopy can be helpful in evaluating paratracheal extension of disease, and if performed as a prelude to definitive transthoracic resection, provides excellent anterior tracheal mobilization. However, it is important not to violate the anticipated planes of resection and compromise the oncologic principles of en bloc surgical resection.

12.3 Pathology

Squamous cell carcinoma and adenoid cystic carcinoma are the two most common tracheal tumors and account for more than two-thirds of all primary tumors of the trachea [19]. Squamous cell carcinoma is classically described as the most common primary tracheal tumor [3, 17, 19]. However, a recent review of seven surgical series shows that adenoid cystic

carcinoma is more common in those patients with surgically treated malignant tracheal tumors [13]. Most likely this is because many squamous cell tumors are unresectable at presentation.

Squamous cell carcinoma of the trachea is usually an exophytic and ulcerated lesion. Multiple lesions can occur and require a thorough tracheobronchial examination by the endoscopist. Squamous cell carcinoma of the trachea is aggressive and spreads to regional lymph nodes and to mediastinal structures. One-third of patients may have mediastinal or pulmonary metastases at the time of diagnosis [19], and 37% were unresectable in a large series reported by GRILLO and MATHISEN [8]. Forty percent of patients who underwent tracheal resection for squamous cell carcinoma at the Massachusetts General Hospital had either a previous history, a concurrent finding, or a subsequent occurrence of a squamous cell carcinoma of the respiratory tract [8].

Adenoid cystic carcinoma, previously known as a cylindroma, originates in the epithelium of mucous glands and is more common in the trachea than in the bronchi [11]. It is usually a well-circumscribed smooth, firm tumor, and is ulcerated only occasionally. The true extension of adenoid cystic carcinoma tends to be greater than is suggested visually due to its tendency to spread along submucosal and perineural planes [20]. These tumors grow slowly and are not prone to early metastasis. Initially adenoid cystic carcinoma may displace rather than invade mediastinal structures [19]. Later they may invade cervical and mediastinal structures and metastasize to cervical and mediastinal lymph nodes as well as lungs, liver, and bone [7, 19].

After squamous cell carcinoma and adenoid cystic carcinoma, the most common tumors of the trachea are carcinoid and mucoepidermoid tumors. However, there is a wide variety of rare tumor types with varying degrees of malignancy and from both epithelial and mesenchymal origins [8]. A list of the pathology of tracheal tumors is shown in Table 12.1.

12.4 Tracheal Resection and Reconstruction

Resection with primary reconstruction is the treatment of choice for nearly all tracheal tumors [8, 9, 11–13, 16, 17]. The prognosis for untreated tracheal tumors is poor, even with benign tumors, due to the risk of airway obstruction, but there is insufficient evidence to make firm generalizations about the natural history of the rare tracheal tumors. In benign tracheal tumors, resection with primary

Table 12.1. Pathology of tracheal tumors

Benign	Malignant
Adenoma	Squamous
Chondroma	Adenoid cystic
Chondroblastoma	Carcinoid
Granular cell tumor	Mucoeopidermoid
Leiomyoma	Adenocarcinoma
Paraganglioma	Adenosquamous
Papillomata	Atypical carcinoid
Vascular malformation	Small cell carcinoma
	Melanoma
	Sarcoma

reconstruction is usually feasible [11]. The heterogeneous group of miscellaneous tracheal primaries treated at the Massachusetts General Hospital by GRILLO and MATHISEN had good results from tracheal resection, with a 2% operative mortality and a 90% disease-free survival of 1–19 years. Many of these tumors were benign or of low-grade malignancy and all these appear to have been cured by complete surgical resection. However, the series did include nine patients with malignant tracheal tumors, three of whom (33%) ultimately died from their primary [8].

Squamous cell carcinoma can be locally aggressive and metastatic at the time of presentation. In Grillo and Mathisen's series of 70 squamous cell carcinomas of the trachea, only 44 patients (63%) were resectable by tracheal resection and reconstruction. In this group, 7/19 (37%) survived more than 5 years free of disease and 13/17 (76%) patients operated on within the past 5 years were alive and disease free, though with insufficient follow-up to be considered cured. Four patients died without disease more than 5 years after surgical resection, to make the disease-free survival at 5 years 11/23 (48%). This is significant since most tumor deaths occurred early, with 8/13 within the first 3 years and 13/13 within 5 years. Six out of eight (75%) patients with positive lymph nodes and four of five (80%) patients with invasive carcinoma at the margin subsequently died with cancer while all patients with carcinoma in situ at the margin were alive and disease-free. There was a 7% operative mortality in this series of resected squamous carcinomas [8].

Results are more difficult to interpret with adenoid cystic carcinoma since this tumor has a tendency towards a long clinical course and late recurrence. In the same series from Massachusetts General Hospital, 5/11 (45%) patients were alive and disease free more than 10 years after resection, and 16/23 (70%) were alive and disease free more than 5 years postoperatively. However, these data are less conclusive than the results with squamous cell carcinoma of the trachea. Four patients died of recurrent adenoid cystic carcinoma more than 10 years after surgical resection and one suffered a recurrence 17 years later [8]. Unlike with the squamous cell carcinomas, the presence of positive margins, positive lymph nodes, or both in adenoid cystic carcinoma has little effect on survival compared to patients with negative margins and nodes. Positive margins are not uncommon given the tendency of adenoid cystic carcinoma to spread submucosally and perineurally, and all of these patients are treated with postoperative radiation. Suture line recurrence is rare, with late recurrence more commonly being metastatic to the lung, liver, or brain [8]. There was an operative mortality of 8/60 (13%) in surgically treated adenoid cystic carcinoma at the Massachusetts General Hospital, but half of these deaths occurred in patients who underwent carinal resections and reconstructions and the other four were a result of staged procedures that have since been abandoned. There was no operative mortality among patients undergoing tracheal resection and reconstruction for adenoid cystic carcinoma [8].

12.5 Radiation Therapy

Radiation has three roles in the treatment of primary tracheal tumors: as primary treatment for cure, as a postoperative adjunct to surgery, and as palliative therapy. Because of the rarity of tracheal tumors, there are few large series in which radiation has been used as primary therapy. Most of the series reporting radiation results include the results of radiation combined with complete or incomplete resection and include the whole spectrum of pathology and a range of radiation doses, making interpretation of the results more difficult. Comparison with surgical results is also difficult since these primary radiation series include surgically resectable and unresectable lesions to varying degrees. Obviously, those weighted towards more advanced disease would be expected to show less encouraging results.

In a review of several series of primary radiation without surgery, local control was obtained in 33%–50% [1, 21, 24]. In squamous cell carcinoma, local control ranged from 11%–46% [22, 23]. The rate of local recurrence for all tumors was 55%–95% [22, 23], resulting in a median survival of 10–26 months [21, 24] and a 5-year survival of 8%–17% [1, 21, 22]. Radiation doses > 60 Gy were significantly more effective at achieving local control than smaller doses [1, 21, 24]. No series had a large enough number of patients with adenoid cystic carcinoma treated with radiation alone to come to any real conclusions regarding its efficacy as definitive therapy. Major morbidity of radiotherapy was reported at 8%–43% [1, 21–24], with a significant number of tracheo-esophageal fistulas (7%–10%) [22–24] and airway obstructions requiring surgery (8%) [1, 22, 24]. Mortality during radiotherapy or as a result of radiotherapy was 8%–13% [21, 22]. All authors concluded that primary surgical resection and reconstruction is the procedure of choice for resectable tracheal tumors [1, 21–25].

GRILLO and MATHISEN compared the results of surgical resection with or without radiation to the results obtained with radiation alone. Of 29 patients with squamous cell carcinoma treated by surgical resection ± radiation, 18 (62%) were alive at 1 year and the median survival was 34 months, while those treated with radiation alone had a 1-year survival of 6% (1/17) and a median survival of 10 months. Patients with adenoid cystic carcinoma had a 1-year survival of 84% (38/45) and a median survival of 118 months after surgical resection ± radiation. One-year survival was 25% (3/12) and median survival was 28 months after primary radiation [8]. Similar results were obtained by Chow at the M.D. Anderson Cancer Center, though with much smaller numbers. Patients treated with surgery and radiation had a median survival of 61 months while those treated with radiation alone had a median survival of 26 months [24]. Clearly these are not randomized trials and patients were usually referred for radiation alone when they were considered unresectable. However, unresectability was often due to longitudinal extent of disease rather than to large bulk of neoplasm [8]. There are no prospective randomized trials to directly compare surgical results with radiation.

Recently, there has been enthusiasm about the preliminary results of fast neutron radiation for the treatment of adenoid cystic carcinomas of the trachea, due to the favorable results with adenoid cystic carcinoma of the salivary glands [26–28]. Early results are encouraging, with a local response rate of 83% and a complete response rate of 60% [26]. However, four of six patients (67%) have died of cancer from 12 to 60 months after neutron radiation, and one of the remaining two patients has an incomplete response, with the single disease-free

survivor having been followed for only 14 months [26]. It does seem clear that neutron radiation has a distinct advantage over photon radiation in cases of adenoid cystic carcinoma [27, 28]. However, these are preliminary studies with small numbers of patients and short follow-up, particularly considering the prolonged course of adenoid cystic carcinoma. Patients with surgically resectable lesions should undergo tracheal resection and reconstruction with adjuvant radiation therapy, reserving high-energy fast neutron beam radiation as an alternative modality for patients with unresectable adenoid cystic carcinoma.

Radiation clearly has an important role as an adjunct to surgery. Usually there are narrow margins at best after tracheal resection for squamous cell carcinoma and adenoid cystic carcinoma given the technical limitations of tracheal reconstruction, the lack of a tracheal prosthesis, and the tendency for adenoid cystic carcinoma to spread along submucosal and perineural planes. Those with the greatest experience in the treatment of these tumors usually recommend postoperative radiation for both squamous cell and adenoid cystic carcinoma, even in the absence of nodal metastases or positive margins [8, 9]. In centers where high-energy fast neutron beam therapy is available this may be adjunctive treatment of choice for adenoid cystic carcinoma.

12.6 Palliation

There are multiple techniques for the palliation of unresectable obstructing tracheal tumors: rigid bronchoscopy with core-out of tumor, CO_2 or Nd:YAG laser vaporization, endotracheal stenting, tracheal T-tubes, tracheostomy, external beam radiation, brachytherapy, cryosurgery, and various combinations of these techniques. Rigid bronchoscopy and core-out has been previously discussed and is expeditious and effective with low morbidity and mortality when performed by experienced therapeutic endoscopists [18]. Several authors advocate laser vaporization for endobronchial debulking, usually combined with mechanical debridement [11, 29–33]. There is a small experience with endobronchial cryotherapy for palliation of endobronchial tumors [11, 34, 35], but it has never become popularized, most likely due to the success of laser vaporization and bronchoscopic core-out [11, 18].

Endobronchial silicone stents, T-tubes, or T-Y tubes can be placed to palliate intrinsic or extrinsic obstructing lesions [36–39] and may be especially effective when combined with endoluminal debulking of the tumor. Stents and T-tubes offer the advantage of long-term palliation when rapid recurrence is expected after core-out or vaporization. They are especially useful for palliation of extrinsic compression that is impossible to relieve by endoscopic methods. Stents and T-tubes also provide airway protection during initiation of external beam radiation, when edema can precipitate acute airway obstruction.

External beam radiation provides palliation for 33%–50% of patients with malignant tracheal tumors, though these patients have a median survival of only 10–26 months [1, 21, 24]. Fast neutron radiation may provide the best palliation for adenoid cystic carcinoma but is available in few centers in the United States [26]. Complications with radiation occur in 8%–43% of patients [1, 21, 24] but it is often the only option for a desperate group of patients with unresectable tracheal tumors. Endobronchial brachytherapy has been used extensively for endobronchial extension or recurrence of bronchogenic carcinoma [40, 41]. The primary advantage is in providing a high localized dose to symptomatic endobronchial extension of disease, particularly when external beam radiation has already been maximized. However, the experience in primary tracheal tumors is very small [42, 43] and so its role in palliation remains unclear. When external beam treatment is limited by the previous doses delivered to the spinal cord, heart, and lungs, endobronchial brachytherapy may provide additional palliation for recurrent tracheobronchial malignancy. There is no significant experience with chemotherapy for tracheal tumors though it may be useful when combined with radiation, as in similar tumors in the head and neck.

12.7 Conclusion

Tracheal tumors are rare and a high index of suspicion is important when a patient presents with dyspnea, stridor, or refractory asthma. Rigid bronchoscopy is critical for detection, diagnosis, surgical planning, relief of acute obstruction, and palliation of tracheal tumors. Resectability is determined by the assessment of local extension and longitudinal extent of tumor. Tracheal resection and reconstruction remains the treatment of choice for nearly all tracheal tumors. Resectable benign tumors are cured by tracheal resection and reconstruction and the results with malignant tumors are dependent on the

histology. The morbidity and mortality of tracheal and carinal resection is acceptable in centers with a large experience in airway surgery.

Radiation is an important adjunct to surgery after resection of squamous and adenoid cystic carcinomas of the trachea. It is also the mainstay of palliation combined with endobronchial techniques of tumor core-out, laser vaporization, and stenting. Patients with unresectable tumors can be offered palliation for months to years through a combination of these techniques, rather than being forced to suffocate from the progression of their tumor.

References

1. Rostom AY, Morgan RL (1978) Results of treating primary tumours of the trachea by irradiation. Thorax 33: 387
2. (1981) Surveillance, epidemiology, and end results. Incidence and mortality data, 1973–1977. In: U.S. Department of Health and Human Services, (Young JL, Percy CL, Asire AJ) Bethesda
3. Houston HE, Payne WS, Harrison EG Jr, Olsen AM (1969) Primary cancers of the trachea. Arch Surg 99: 132–140
4. Karlan MS, Livingston PA, Baker DC (1973) Diagnosis of tracheal tumors. Ann Otol Rhinol Laryngol 82: 790–799
5. Eschapasse H (1974) Les tumeurs tracheales primitives: traitement chirurgical. Rev Fr Malad Resp 2: 425
6. Grillo HC (1978) Tracheal tumors: surgical management. Ann Thorac Surg 26: 112–125
7. Grillo HC (1982) Carinal reconstruction. Ann Thorac Surg 34: 356–373
8. Grillo HC, Mathisen DJ (1990) Primary tracheal tumors: treatment and results. Ann Thorac Surg 49: 69–77
9. Pearson FG, Todd TRJ, Cooper JD (1984) Experience with primary neoplasms of the trachea. J Thorac Cardiovasc Surg 88: 511–516
10. Perelman M, Koroleva N (1980) Surgery of the trachea. World J Surg 4: 583–593
11. Perelman MI, Koroleva NS (1987) Primary tumors of the trachea. In: Grillo HC, Eschapasse H (eds) International trends in general thoracic surgery, vol 2. Saunders, Philadelphia, pp 91–106
12. Xu LT, Sun ZF, Li ZJ, Wu LH, Zhang ZY, Yu ZQ (1987) Clinical and pathologic characteristics in patients with tracheobronchial tumor: report of 50 patients. Ann Thorac Surg 43: 276–278
13. Allen MS (1993) Malignant tracheal tumors. Mayo Clin Proc 68: 680–684
14. Weber AL, Grillo HC (1978) Tracheal tumors: radiologic, clinical, and pathological evaluation. Adv Otorhinolaryngol 24: 170–176
15. Grillo HC (1983) Tracheal tumors: diagnosis and management. In: Choi NC, Grillo HC (eds) Thoracic oncology. Raven Press, New York, pp 271–278
16. Eschapasse H (1987) Primary tumors of the trachea. In: Grillo HC, Eschapasse H (eds) International trends in general thoracic surgery, vol 2. Saunders, Philadelphia, pp 107–110

17. Pairolero PC (1989) Benign and malignant neoplasms of the trachea. In: Roth JA, Ruckdeschel JC, Weisenburger TH (eds) Thoracic oncology. Saunders, Philadelphia, pp 513–519

18. Mathisen DJ, Grillo HC (1989) Endoscopic relief of malignant airway obstruction. Ann Thorac Surg 48: 469–475

19. Grillo HC (1990) Congenital lesions, neoplasms, and injuries of the trachea. In: Sabiston DC, Spencer FC (eds) Surgery of the chest, 5th edn. Saunders, Philadelphia, pp 335–371

20. Pearson FG, Thompson DW, Weissberg D, Simpson WJK, Kergin FG (1974) Adenoid cystic carcinoma of the trachea. Ann Thorac Surg 18: 16–29

21. Fields JN, Rigaud G, Emami BN (1989) Primary tumors of the trachea: results of radiation therapy. Cancer 63: 2429–2433

22. Manninen MP, Pukander JS, Flander MK, Laippla PJ, Huhtala HSA, Karma PH (1993) Treatment of primary tracheal carcinoma in Finland in 1967–1985. Acta Oncol 32: 277–282

23. Cheung AYC (1989) Radiotherapy for primary carcinoma of the trachea. Radiother Oncol 14: 279–285

24. Chow DC, Komaki R, Libshitz HI, Mountain CF, Ellerbroek N (1993) Treatment of primary neoplasms of the trachea: the role of radiation therapy. Cancer 71: 2946–2952

25. Ampil FL (1986) Primary malignant tracheal neoplasms: case reports and literature radiotherapy review. J Surg Oncol 33: 20–23

26. Saroja KR (1993) Treatment of tracheal tumors with high energy fast neutron radiation. Oncology 7: 16, 21–22

27. Laramore GE, Krall JM, Griffin TW et al. (1993) Neutron vs photon irradiation for unresectable salivary gland tumors: final report of an RTOG-MRC randomized clinical trial. Int J Radiat Oncol Biol Phys 27: 235–240

28. Buchholz TA, Shimotakahara SG, Weymuller EA, Laramore GE, Griffin TW (1993) Neutron radiation for adenoid cystic carcinoma of the head and neck. Arch Octolaryngol Head Neck Surg 119: 747–752

29. McDougall JC, Cortese DA (1983) Neodymium- YAG laser of malignant airway obstruction: a preliminary report. Mayo Clin Proc 58: 35–39

30. Shapshay SM, Dumon JF, Beamis JF (1985) Endoscopic treatment of tracheobronchial malignancy: experience with the Nd: YAG and CO_2 lasers in 506 operations. Otolaryngol Head Neck Surg 93: 205–210

31. Cavaliere S, Foccoli P, Farina PL (1988) Nd: YAG laser bronchoscopy: a five-year experience with 1,396 applications in 1,000 patients. Chest 94: 15–21

32. Dumon JF, Reboud E, Garbe L, Aucomte F, Meric B (1982) Treatment of tracheobronchial lesions by laser photoresection. Chest 81: 278–284

33. McElvein RB, Zorn GL Jr (1984) Indications, results, and complications of bronchoscopic carbon dioxide laser therapy. Ann Surg 199: 522–525

34. Marasso A, Gallo E, Massaglia GM, Onoscuri M, Bernardi V (1993) Cryosurgery in bronchoscopic treatment of tracheobronchial stenosis: indications, limits, personal experience. Chest 103: 472–474

35. Rodgers BM, Talbert JL (1978) Clinical application of endotracheal cryotherapy. J Pediatr Surg 13: 662–668

36. Orlowski TM (1987) Palliative intubation of the tracheobronchial tree. J Thorac Cardiovasc Surg 94: 343–348

37. Cooper JD, Pearson FG, Patterson GA, Todd TRJ, Ginsberg RJ, Goldberg M, Waters P (1989) Use of silicone stents in the management of airway problems. Ann Thorac Surg 47: 371–378

38. Landa L (1987) The tracheal T-tube: in tracheal surgery. In: Grillo HC, Eschapasse H (eds) International trends in general thoracic surgery, vol 2. Saunders, Philadelphia, pp 124–132

39. Keszler P (1987) The tracheal T-tube: for indwelling intubation as an alternative management method. In: Grillo HC, Eschapasse H (eds) International trends in general thoracic surgery, vol 2. Saunders, Philadelphia, pp 133–137

40. Raju PI, Roy T, McDonald RD et al. (1993) IR-192, low dose rate endobronchial brachytherapy in the treatment of malignant airway obstruction. Int J Radiat Oncol Biol Phys 27: 677–680

41. Nori D, Allison R, Kaplan B, Samala E, Osian A, Karbowitz S (1993) High dose-rate intraluminal irradiation in bronchogenic carcinoma: technique and results. Chest 104: 1006–1011

42. Chin HW, DeMeester T, Chin RY, Boman B (1991) Endobronchial adenoid cystic carcinoma. Chest 100: 1464–1465

43. Percarpio B, Price JC, Murphy P (1978) Endotracheal irradiation of adenoid cystic carcinoma of the trachea. Radiology 128: 209–210

13 Mesenchymal Tumors of the Mediastinum

JONATHAN SOMERS and L. PENFIELD FABER

CONTENTS

JONATHAN SOMERS, M.D., Assistant Professor of Surgery, Rush Medical College; Assistant Attending in Cardiovascular and Thoracic Surgery, Rush-Presbyterian-St. Luke's Medical Center, 1725 W. Harrison St., Chicago, IL 60612, USA
L. PENFIELD FABER, M.D., Professor of Surgery, Rush Medical College; Chief of General Thoracic Section and Senior Attending, Department of Cardiovascular and Thoracic Surgery, Rush-Presbyterian-St. Luke's Medical Center, 1725 W. Harrison St., Chicago, IL 60612, USA

13.1 Introduction

Mesenchymal tumors of the mediastinum are a heterogeneous group of benign and malignant neoplasms originating from a variety of tissues. They are uncommon, accounting for only 6%–8% of all mediastinal masses [1–9]. They are slightly more common in children and constitute 10% or more of mediastinal tumors in younger age groups [8].

These tumors are typically classified by their tissue of origin (Table 13.1). Differences in opinion exist as to whether or not tumors of thymic tissue should be included in this classification; however, most categorize these tumors under the separate grouping of mediastinal thymic tumors [6–8, 10]. We have chosen to follow a similar course and have not included thymolipomas or thymoliposarcomas in this discussion. Similarly, because of common tissue origin we have included leiomyomas and leiomyosarcomas in our discussion of tumors of muscle origin, and not in the discussion of tumors of blood vessel origin despite the fact that these tumors are most commonly associated with the great vessels in the mediastinum.

Nearly half of all mesenchymal neoplasms of the mediastinum are tumors of endothelium (lymphatic or vascular). Tumors of lymphatic origin are the more common and the majority of these are benign. Overall, however, 55% of mediastinal mesenchymal tumors are malignant, with a somewhat higher incidence of malignancy in children [1,4].

Symptoms and findings associated with this diverse group of tumors vary greatly with size, location within the mediastinum, and degree of malignancy. For example, lipomas of the mediastinum are more often than not discovered incidentally on chest x-ray, while liposarcomas usually present with symptoms of painful or respiratory difficulty. Children, with a higher incidence of malignant tumors, are more likely than adults to present with symptoms.

Table 13.1. Classification of mesenchymal tumors of mediastinum

Tumors of lymph vessel origin
  Lymphangioma
  Lymphangiomatosis
  Lymphangiomyoma
Tumors of blood vessel origin
  Hemangioma
  Hemangioendothelioma
  Angiosarcoma
Tumors of pericyte origin
  Hemangiopericytoma (benign and malignant)
Tumors of adipose tissue origin
  Lipoma
  Lipomatosis
  Lipoblastomatosis
  Liposarcoma
Tumors of fibrous tissue origin
  Fibromatosis
  Fibrosarcoma
  Malignant fibrous histiocytoma
Tumors of muscular origin
  Rhabdomyoma
  Rhabdomyosarcoma
  Leiomyoma
  Leiomyosarcoma
Tumors of skeletal tissue origin
  Chondroma
  Chondrosarcoma
Tumors of pluripotential mesenchyme
  Mesenchymoma (benign and malignant)
  Synovial sarcoma
Other mesenchymal tumors
  Solitary fibrous tumor
  Meningioma
  Chordoma
  Granular cell tumor
  Mediastinal xanthoma

13.2 Tumors of Lymph Vessel Origin

13.2.1 Lymphangioma

Lymphangiomas are benign, slow-growing tumors composed of lymphatic vessels. Less than 1% are confined to the mediastinum [11]. They are categorized as simple, cavernous, or cystic depending on the histologic size of their cystic spaces [12]. Simple tumors have capillary size lymph channels. Cavernous tumors, on the other hand, have larger spaces forming a sponge-like mass. Cystic hygromas typically have large, multiloculated spaces filled with chyle.

There are two distinct types of mediastinal lymphangiomas: the rare primary lesion that is confined to the mediastinum and occurs almost exclusively in adults, and the far more common infantile type that extends from the neck into the mediastinum [13]. Approximately 10% of all infantile lymphangiomas extend into the mediastinum, but rare cases of purely mediastinal cystic hygromas have been reported [14]. Both types are equally distributed between males and females and have a small percentage associated with such diverse abnormalities as concurrent hemangiomas, chylothorax (secondary to spontaneous or traumatic rupture of the tumor), disappearing bone disease, and multiple lesions involving other organs (see Sect. 13.2.2).

There is great variation in the pathology of these tumors. They may or may not be well circumscribed, and they can vary in size from less than a centimeter to giant lesions filling most of the thorax. They are grayish in color and have a sponge-like quality with cystic spaces filled with chyle. The presence of chyle is usually noted at the time of resection. Histologically, they are composed of multiple lymphatic vessels of varying size lined by endothelial cells. They are differentiated from hemangiomas both by the presence of chyle and by lymphoid infiltrates [10]. Immunocytochemical techniques can also be used to distinguish between lymphatic and vascular tumors. This testing is based on the fact that the endothelial cells lining lymphatics lack the intracytoplasmic factor VIII found in vascular endothelial cells. Mixed forms (lymphangiohemangioma) have been reported but are exceedingly rare [15].

Most mediastinal lymphangiomas in adults are asymptomatic and found on routine chest radiographs. Rarely, they present with symptoms of dyspnea or heart failure secondary to atrial or ventricular compression [11]. Children with mediastinal spread of a cervical lymphangioma often present with visible disfigurement of the lower neck, and less commonly with symptoms of tracheal or vascular compression [10–17]. Infrequently, the lesions can become infected and present with signs of inflammation.

Chest radiographs usually demonstrate a smooth, lobulated, or round noncalcified mass in the mediastinum (Fig. 13.1). BROWN reported roughly 30% to be located in the anteroinferior mediastinum, with another third in the posterior mediastinum and the remainder in the superior mediastinum [11]. Computed tomography (CT) is very helpful in demonstrating the cystic nature of these lesions, and may establish the diagnosis. PILLA et al. described four characteristic CT findings of these lesions: (a) smooth and well circumscribed without invasion

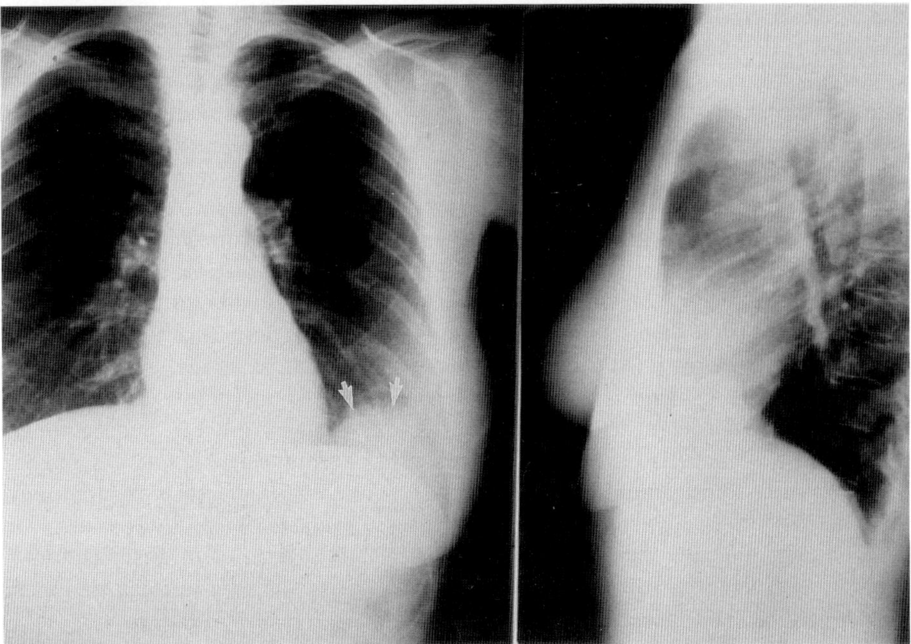

Fig. 13.1. Radiographs of a smooth, rounded appearing lymphangioma (*arrows*) in the mid-mediastinum

of adjacent tissues, (b) displacement or envelopment of normal structures, (c) absence of calcifications and (d) varying attenuation values [18]. Magnetic resonance images typically reveal thin-walled, multiloculated cystic masses of high signal intensity [19]. Depending on whether or not there is communication between the tumor and the thoracic duct, lymphangiography may reveal accumulation of contrast medium in the tumor, or extravasation of contrast medium into the pleural space in cases of spontaneous or traumatic rupture of a mediastinal lymphangioma. However, lymphangiography is rarely used and is usually not required for diagnosis.

Complete surgical excision, when possible, is the treatment of choice. Freedom from local recurrence following initial complete excision of anterior mediastinal lesions in adults is the usual situation. However, in cases of infantile cystic hygromas of the cervical region that extend into the superior mediastinum, complete excision often requires extensive dissection. Although local recurrence may occur following limited resection, this is preferable to injury to important neural or vascular structures from a more extensive resection. In these situations, repeat conservative resection is advised, and continued recurrences, fortunately, are unusual. Treatment with radiation has been marginally successful, but may be associated with malignant transformation of the tumor and is recommended only after other therapies for persistent chylothorax have failed [16, 20]. Sclerotherapy has been unsuccessfully attempted with multiple agents and is also not recommended.

Multiple treatments for chylothorax associated with mediastinal lymphangioma have been proposed. These therapies include simple conservative management with tube thoracostomy, pleuroperitoneal shunting, and ligation of the thoracic duct. All have been used with variable success [21–25]. Our preference for treatment of persistent chylothorax that does not respond to conservative therapy (tube thoracostomy and parenteral nutrition) is ligation of the thoracic duct via a right thoracotomy.

13.2.2 Lymphangiomatosis

The presence of multiple lymphangiomas arising in both somatic and visceral sites is termed "lymphangiomatosis." This disease is a congenital systemic lymphatic malformation and is manifested predominantly in children under age 20 [26–28]. It is frequently associated with chylothorax, lymphopenia, and hypogammaglobulinemia. Persistent chylothorax is common and is responsible for the high mortality associated with this disease. Additionally, these lesions have a strong tendency to extend into adjacent tissues and may not be resectable. Treatment consists in surgical correction of the chylothorax and resection of the mediastinal tumor when possible.

13.2.3 Lymphangiomyomatosis

Lymphangiomyomatosis is a rare condition that affects only females of reproductive age. It is characterized by proliferation of lymph vessels and smooth muscle in the lung, retroperitoneum, and mediastinum. These tumors may result from multiple hamartomas [29–33]. On pathologic examination these lesions are lobulated, red-gray, and spongelike, with interconnected endothelial-lined spaces surrounded by fascicles of smooth muscle [10]. Small airway obstruction can be noted on examination of the lung where the muscle fascicles surround interalveolar vessels, causing septal widening and small airway compression. Symptoms include dyspnea and hemoptysis, secondary to lung parenchymal involvement. Dyspnea may also result from spontaneous unilateral or bilateral chylothorax. Isolated lymphangiomyomas of the mediastinum are often asymptomatic and carry a good prognosis. Conversely, those women with pulmonary involvement usually die of respiratory complications within 10 years of initial diagnosis.

Diagnosis is usually made by biopsy of mediastinal lymph nodes or lung nodules. Occasionally, lymphangiograms are done and demonstrate lymph vessel ectasia and obstruction of major ducts suggestive of this lesion. Treatment is again oriented towards relief of the chylothorax. All of the methods described previously have been attempted. Progesterone treatment has been reported to be useful as well [29]. Bilateral oophorectomy has been recommended for those patients with extensive pulmonary involvement. Lung transplantation has also recently been described for this situation [10].

13.3 Tumors of Blood Vessel Origin

With slightly more than 100 cases reported in the literature, tumors of blood vessel origin are rare, constituting less than 1% of all mediastinal tumors. Three-fourths of these tumors are benign and the vast majority are either cavernous or capillary hemangiomas [34]. The remaining 25%, including hemangioendotheliomas and angiosarcomas, are malignant. Although hemangiopericytomas are sometimes included in this category because of their occurrence around pericapillary arterioles, we have chosen to discuss them separately because their origin is from pericytes and not from endothelial cells.

Mediastinal tumors derived from blood vessels are distributed equally among males and females, and are found in all age groups. Cavernous hemangiomas constitute the majority of these tumors in children [35]. Symptoms are present in 33%–45% of patients, and are usually related to invasion of mediastinal structures [34]. Malignant lesions almost always cause symptoms; these include cough, stridor, dyspnea, hoarseness, chest pain, dysphasia, Horner's syndrome, superior vena cava syndrome, and neurologic manifestations from cord compression. Asymptomatic patients are usually found to have a mediastinal mass on routine chest films. Rarely, these lesions are discovered as part of a workup for diffuse hemangiomatosis, as seen in the Osler-Weber-Rendu and Klippel-Trenaunay syndromes.

13.3.1 Hemangioma

As stated above, these tumors account for 90% of all mediastinal vascular tumors and the vast majority are benign. As with lymphangiomas, these tumors are classified according to the size of their vascular spaces into cavernous, capillary, and venous hemangiomas [36]. Cavernous hemangiomas are the most common type and are composed of large vascular spaces with smooth muscle walls and a stroma that is edematous and has myxomatous areas containing stellate cells [10]. The vascular spaces or blood vessels are lined with flattened endothelial cells. An unusual variant of this tumor, termed hamartomatous hemangioma or angiomyoma, is characterized by a prominent smooth muscle component [7, 37–45]. Capillary hemangiomas are characterized by a mass of capillaries with prominent endothelial cells. These account for approximately 15% of mediastinal hemangiomas. The venous type of tumor is very rare and is composed of a mass of thick-walled vessels, with a large amount of smooth muscle cells in the vessel walls. Grossly, these tumors all appear as well-circumscribed, soft, red masses that exude blood and deflate and sectioning. As noted previously, they are distinguished from lymphangiomas on the basis of blood-filled vessels (as opposed to the chyle-filled vessels in lymphangiomas) and, if necessary, by immunocytochemical techniques.

Diagnosis of these tumors is usually suggested by CT or magnetic resonance imaging (MRI). Plain films of the chest demonstrate the location of the lesion in the mediastinum and may demonstrate phleboliths in up to 10% of patients. Phleboliths are considered diagnostic if present, but in a recent series of 15 patients none were found on plain films [34]. CT scan is useful in demonstrating phleboliths and also the exact location and extent of mediastinal invasion. Typically, these lesions appear as homogeneous, solid masses on CT scan with attenuation figures of 30 HU. These lesions may or may not enhance with intravenous contrast administration, but attenuation is distinctly different than that of adjacent vascular structures. Dynamic CT scanning following intravenous administration of iodinated contrast usually demonstrates papillary enhancement with peripheral puddling of contrast medium and may be the most accurate single diagnostic study. Several reports of MRI of these lesions preliminarily indicate that while the vascular nature of the tumor may be revealed, the MR appearance is not specific for hemangiomas [46–48]. Angiography is not useful for diagnosis since these lesions do not opacify with arterial administration of contrast medium. Venography may rarely identify these lesions but it will most likely be replaced by dynamic CT scanning [34].

Treatment of symptomatic tumors is complete surgical excision when possible [34–45]. The best approach, either posterolateral thoracotomy or median sternotomy, is dictated by the location and extent of the tumor. Complete excision is possible 50% of the time, and is usually limited by infiltration of adjacent vascular, neural, or bony mediastinal structures. Partial resection using cautery and extensive suture-ligation usually can be performed without excessive hemorrhage, and is recommended. Nevertheless, a single report of postoperative exsanguination following partial excision has led some authors to recommend complete excision only [40]. These authors successfully managed a patient with a tumor invading the superior vena cava with complete excision and replacement of the cava using a prosthetic graft. However, because these tumors do not undergo malignant transformation and because recurrence after partial excision is uncommon, conservative resection is advised in cases where total excision appears hazardous.

13.3.2 Hemangioendothelioma

The term "hemangioendothelioma" is used to describe three subtypes of tumors that are intermediate between benign hemangiomas and malignant angio-sarcomas: (1) epithelioid hemangioendothelioma, (2) spindle cell hemangioendothelioma, and (3) the "Dabska" tumor. However, all mediastinal cases reported in the literature are referred to as epithelioid hemangioendotheliomas, and whether or not types 2 and 3 are included in this description is not specified [49–51].

Epithelioid hemangioendothelioma is a rare tumor of low-grade malignancy derived from endothelial cells and only a handful of cases of isolated mediastinal tumors exist in the literature. More commonly, these tumors are found in the soft tissues of the extremities, the liver, bone, submandibular region, and pulmonary parenchyma. In the lung they typically occur in young women as multiple bilateral nodules less than 2 cm in diameter.

The degree of malignancy of these lesions is judged clinically on the presence of encapsulation and local infiltration of adjacent tissues. More than 50% of mediastinal lesions arise from large veins such as the innominate or jugular veins [36, 50], and on examination they appear as a fusiform expansion of the vessel or as a solid mass enveloping the vessel [49]. They generally occur in the anterior and posterior mediastinum. Of the 19 cases cited by Toursarkissian and associates, six occurred in the posterior mediastinum and these were all in children. There appears to be no sex or age predilection.

On sectioning, these tumors appear red-white and can fill the involved vessel. Unlike hemangiomas or angiosarcomas, they are rarely hemorrhagic. Microscopically, these lesions are composed of small nests or cords of rounded or spindled endothelial cells with an epithelioid quality [50]. These cells are embedded within a basophilic myxoid matrix resembling hyaline cartilage that is rich in sulfated acid mucins. The large, well-formed vascular channels found in hemangiomas are not present. Immunocytochemistry and electron microscopy are helpful in confirming the endothelial nature of these tumors.

Although the lack of experience with isolated mediastinal lesions prohibits clear-cut recommendations for treatment, the larger experience with soft tissue epithelioid hemangioendotheliomas may suggest some therapeutic guidelines. In soft tissues, these tumors have a high rate of both local recurrence and metastasis, and wide surgical excision with lymphadenectomy is advised [36, 49]. While the degree of metaplasia and pleomorphism may indicate the malignant behavior of these tumors, histologically benign lesions may behave in a clinically malignant manner, and therefore wide excision with resection of regional lymph nodes is the primary goal in treatment. Intraoperative frozen-section pathologic studies may be useful in obtaining margins free of tumor. The best surgical approach is again dictated by the location of the lesion. Adjuvant radiation and chemotherapy they have advocated for the malignant-appearing tumors, although studies evaluating their efficacy are lacking. Metastases and local recurrences should be treated with surgical excision, as patients with both have been cured [49].

13.3.3 Angiosarcoma

Angiosarcomas are rare malignant tumors of blood vessels that can develop in a variety of locations, including bones, viscera, and soft tissues. In the mediastinum they are almost always tumors of the heart (more specifically the right atrium), although cases involving the superior vena cava, innominate vein, left atrium, and pericardium have been reported. Exposure to vinyl chloride monomer has been recognized as a risk factor for development of these tumors.

Angiosarcomas are invasive, ill-defined masses arising from major blood vessels that microscopically are formed of anastomosing vascular channels lined by atypical endothelium. The endothelial cells are pleomorphic and multinucleated and, as with all blood vessel tumors, stain positive for factor VIII-related antigen.

Primary mediastinal angiosarcomas (i.,e., those arising from the venae cavae or innominate vein) are so rare that few conclusions can be drawn from the isolated reports in the literature. Nevertheless, rough guidelines may be inferred from experience with angiosarcomas arising elsewhere.

ABRATT and associates reported a case in which the tumor arose from the superior vena cava [52]. The vessel was not obstructed and the patient presented with intermittent right-sided chest pain. Chest films demonstrated a right anterior mediastinal mass, and at operation he was found to have a 7-cm-diameter mass that arose from superior vena cava. The superior vena cava was resected and reconstruction was by means of separate Dacron grafts from the left and right innominate veins to the right atrium. This patient received postoperative adjuvant radiation therapy to the upper mediastinum and remained well with no evidence of recurrence or metastasis 2 years after treatment. The usefulness of postoperative radiation therapy has been established for angiosarcomas arising elsewhere in the body and

it should be considered in the treatment of mediastinal tumors.

MILLER and co-workers reported a case of primary angiosarcoma that arose in the innominate vein of a middle-aged female who presented with symptoms of chest pain and signs related to obstruction of the innominate vein [53]. Chest films demonstrated an anterior mediastinal mass and venogram demonstrated complete occlusion of the innominate vein. Surgery was performed through a median sternotomy, and excision of the tumor was carried out without reconstruction of the innominate vein. No adjuvant therapy was given and the patient was free of tumor after 8 years.

In summary, while the experience with angiosarcomas of the mediastinum is very limited, wide surgical excision is indicated and routine postoperative radiation therapy should be strongly considered.

13.4 Tumors of Pericyte Origin

13.4.1 Hemangiopericytoma

Hemangiopericytomas are rare, solitary tumors that arise from cells that surround pericapillary arterioles. They are frequently included in discussions of tumors of blood vessel origin despite the fact that they are not endothelial-derived tumors. Both the benign and the malignant form have been reported to occur as isolated, primary mediastinal lesions, and grossly both forms appear as soft, gray-white masses. The benign form occurs more commonly in the anterior mediastinum and is well circumscribed, while the malignant form usually develops in the posterior mediastinum and is less well encapsulated. Symptoms are more common with the malignant form and are usually related to infiltration or compression of adjacent structures [16, 36, 54].

Histologically, these lesions are highly vascularized and are composed of irregular endothelial-lined spaces arranged in a classic branched or "stag horn" pattern. The cells can form solid areas but are not aligned in the fascicles typical of other mesenchymal spindle cell tumors. Reticulin stains reveal that the cells are outside the vascular channels. Malignancy is best indicated by the infiltrative growth pattern and/or metastasis.

Diagnosis is usually made at surgery, as CT scan does not reliably distinguish these tumors. Treatment is wide excision of the lesion with resection of local lymph nodes. Adriamycin has been reported to be useful in treating the malignant form of this tumor.

13.5 Tumors of Adipose Tissue Origin

13.5.1 Lipoma

Lipomas are benign lesions that account for 1% of mediastinal tumors [9]. They can occur singly or as multiple rounded and well circumscribed lesions in the mediastinum. They vary greatly in size, and can reach gigantic proportions. Most occur in the anterior compartment but middle and posterior mediastinal lipomas have been reported. They can extend through the chest wall through an intercostal space, or into the spinal canal via an intervertebral foramen.

On pathologic examination they are encapsulated soft yellow masses composed of lobules of mature fat [55, 56]. In contrast to the lipomas in adults, lipomas in children occasionally show some mitotic activity and mild cytologic atypia [16].

Symptoms are unusual and are secondary to compression of mediastinal structures or lung. Dyspnea is the most commonly cited symptom. On chest films, these lesions can simulate cardiomegaly, pleural effusions or hilar masses (Fig. 13.2), but CT scan allows accurate identification because of uniform and characteristic low density [57, 58]. They can usually be distinguished by CT scan from thymolipomas, which are bilobate, and from liposarcomas, which have higher density and less well-defined borders.

These lesions are benign and are easily excised, except in the unusual situation where they extend into the spinal canal. This occurrence is demonstrated by preoperative CT or MRI and requires neurosurgical or orthopedic consultation. Complete excision is curative.

13.5.2 Lipomatosis

Unlike the mediastinal lipoma, lipomatosis is characterized by the diffuse accumulation of unencapsulated mediastinal fat. It is associated with obesity, corticosteroid ingestion, and Cushing's syndrome, and occurs in all age groups. As with mediastinal lipoma, the lesion is composed of mature adult fat cells with no microscopic evidence of atypia or mitotic activity. It is a fairly common cause of diffuse mediastinal widening on chest x-ray in patients with Cushing's syndrome, and occurs more commonly in the anterior compartment [59–62]. Diagnosis is easily made in the obese or cushingoid

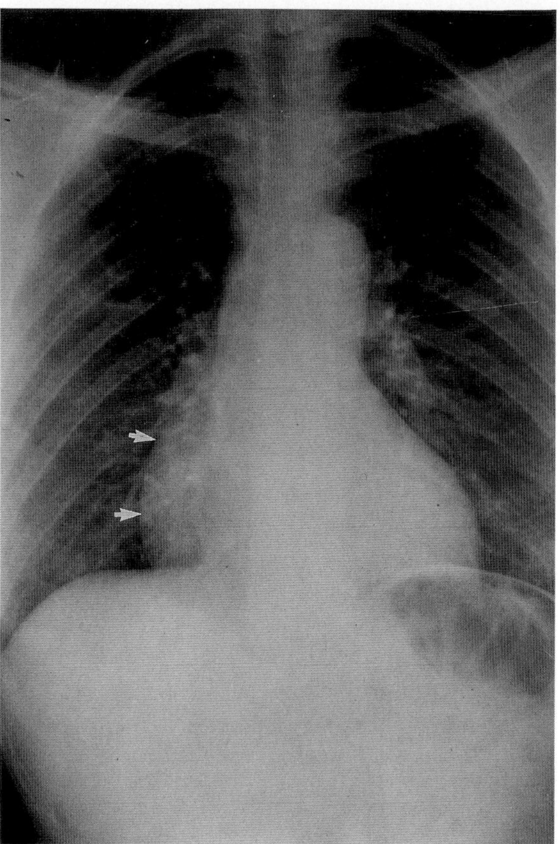

Fig. 13.2. Radiograph of a smooth, rounded appearing anterior mediastinal lipoma (*arrows*) adjacent to the right heart border

patient with CT scan. No treatment is required for this benign and incidentally discovered lesion.

13.5.3 Lipoblastoma and Lipoblastomatosis

Lipoblastomas are rare tumors composed of lobular immature fat with lipoblasts. They occur only in children less than 3 years of age. Approximately 70% of these tumors arise in the limbs. The remainder arise in the mediastinum, neck, axilla, and prevertebral soft tissues [57, 63, 64]. These tumors tend to grow more rapidly than other fat-containing tumors.

On sectioning they are soft and yellow-gray in color. Histologically, they are benign. When well encapsulated, they are referred to as "lipoblastomas." Less well encapsulated lesions that infiltrate surrounding tissues are part of the process of "lipoblastomatosis." The stroma of both types has abundant mucoid material [10]. The lipoblasts can present as stellate, spindle, or polygonal shaped cells with unilocular intracytoplasmic single vacuoles.

Symptoms are secondary to compression and invasion of adjacent tissues. Invasion of the trachea has been reported and can cause respiratory distress and asphyxia. The more invasive forms of these tumors associated with lipoblastomatosis are more commonly symptomatic and are more likely to recur after surgical excision. CT scanning demonstrates a low-density mediastinal mass suggestive of fat. Ultrasound is reported to be useful in diagnosis, demonstrating an echogenic mass with well-defined inner hypoechoic areas representing the myxoid matrix [65–67].

Metastasis has not been reported and treatment by complete excision is curative.

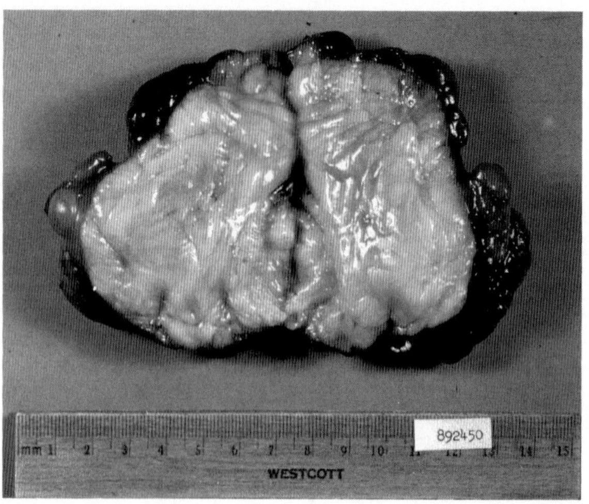

Fig. 13.3. Photograph of a mediastinal liposarcoma on cut section

13.5.4 Liposarcoma

Liposarcomas are uncommon malignant tumors, with slightly more than 50 cases in the available literature [68–72]. Most of these reports describe isolated mediastinal tumors and most occurred in patients of middle age; these lesions are rarely described in children [73]. No specific risk factors for this tumor have been identified. Recently, a case of primary mediastinal liposarcoma has been reported in a patient infected with the human immunodeficiency virus [74].

These tumors tend to be large and lobulated with ill-defined borders. They frequently infiltrate and compress adjacent mediastinal structures. The majority of affected patients are symptomatic, and most present with dyspnea, tachypnea, cough, or wheezing. Many present with constant pain or "pressure" within the thorax. Weight loss is not uncommon.

On gross examination, these tumors are large, unencapsulated but well circumscribed; they are soft, mucoid, and yellow-gray, with focal areas of hemorrhage and necrosis (Fig. 13.3). On occasion liposarcomas can grow to a massive size; LACEY and PETCH reported a tumor weighing 7 kg [75]. Histologically, liposarcomas are categorized into one of the four types: well differentiated, myxoid, pleomorphic, and round cell. The well-differentiated type is the least aggressive form, followed by the myxoid type. Round cell and pleomorphic liposarcomas are more malignant tumors, often presenting with metastasis to lungs and bones at the time of diagnosis. All types contain focal areas of necrosis and varying amounts of malignant lipoblasts with round or oval

hyperchromatic nuclei and foamy cytoplasm. Ultimate identification (and prognosis) is dependent on the presence and number of the malignant lipoblasts, and well-differentiated tumors with few malignant lipoblasts may be difficult to diagnose. Immunocytochemistry is not helpful in identification. They are characterized by the presence of S-100 protein and vimentin.

Radiologically, these tumors present as large, moderately well circumscribed masses that have a density greater than fat but less than water (Fig. 13.4). This finding on CT scan is useful for differentiating these tumors from other tumors of fat.

The optimal treatment for these lesions is complete surgical excision. However, this is often not possible because of extensive infiltration of adjacent mediastinal structures. Incomplete resection has been used in these situations but leads to early recurrence. Radiation therapy is not beneficial. Chemotherapy may be of some benefit in reducing the size of the tumor, but experience is limited.

Prognosis of these lesions is dependent on tumor-type and the presence of pseudo-encapsulation. Tumors with pseudo-encapsulation are usually of the less malignant variety and are more apt to be excised completely. These tumors carry a much better prognosis. The presence of metastasis, associated with the more aggressive types, indicates a grave prognosis. Similarly, all patients who present with superior vena caval obstruction succumb to the disease in less than 2 years.

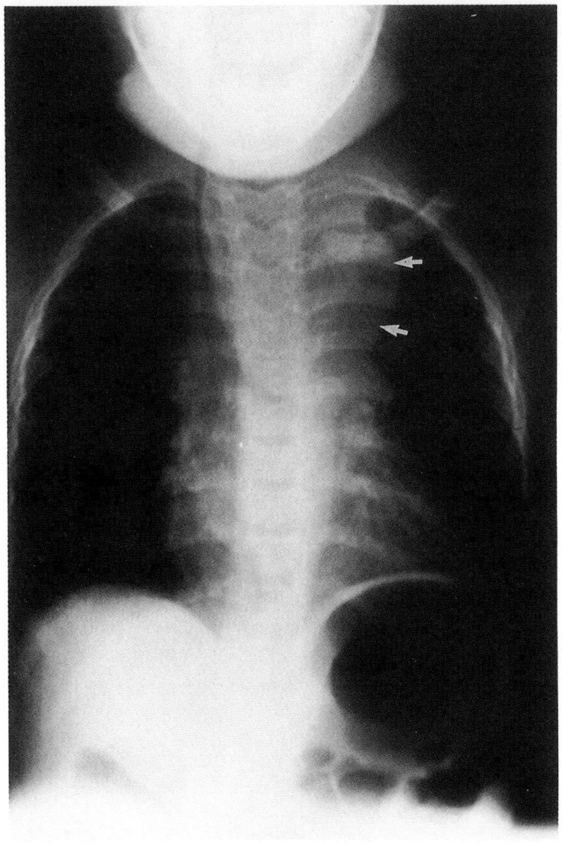

Fig. 13.4. Radiograph of a liposarcoma (*arrows*) in the left, upper, anterior mediastinum

13.6 Tumors of Fibrous Tissue Origin

13.6.1 Fibromatosis

Fibromatosis is characterized by the growth of ill-circumscribed tumors composed of dense masses of collagen and fibroblasts. Also referred to as extraabdominal fibromatosis or extraabdominal desmoid tumors, controversy exists as to whether this condition is a distinct disease process. Some consider these lesions to represent a normal result of the inflammatory response associated with granulomatous disease, while other question whether these "fibromas" really represent benign fibrous mesotheliomas or cases of sclerosing mediastinitis [76–77]. The etiology of this condition is similarly obscure when it affects other areas of the body, such as occurs with palmar fibromatosis (Dupuytren's contracture), or when it affects retroperitoneal structures, as occurs in retroperitoneal fibrosis. In any event,

this condition is distinctly rare in the mediastinum. In their classic paper, PACHTER and LATTES reported only three cases [6].

Grossly, the tumor is dense and white and resembles scar tissue. Histologically, it is composed of rare spindle-shaped fibroblasts surrounded by dense hyalinized collagen. There is infiltration of adjacent tissues of the mediastinum, and resection can be difficult.

Symptoms are related to compression of adjacent structures. Diagnosis is suggested but not confirmed by CT scanning. Symptoms warrant surgical excision, which can be quite difficult if extensive infiltration of mediastinal structures has occurred. Recurrence has been reported after incomplete excision [78]. Other proposed methods of treatment include high-dose radiation as well as hormonal and steroid drug therapy [78–81].

13.6.2 Fibrosarcoma

Fibrosarcomas are rare in the mediastinum. A recent review of the literature could document only 36 cases, and the question has been raised as to whether some of these reported cases were misclassified [16, 82]. Malignant fibrous histiocytoma, leiomyosarcoma, peripheral nerve sheath tumors, and mesotheliomas are examples of tumors mistaken for fibrosarcoma. Most of the patients described have been of middle age. There does not appear to be any sex predilection. Most patients present with symptoms of cough, dyspnea, or dysphagia. Symptoms are related to tumor size, and some very large tumors have been reported. Interestingly, large tumors may be associated with hypoglycemia [82–84]. Although the etiology of the hypoglycemia is unclear, some speculate the tumor may release insulin-like agents that inhibit gluconeogenesis [77].

On chest x-ray, fibrosarcomas are lobulated masses with ill-defined borders that frequently invade adjacent structures, including ribs and vertebral bodies. CT and MRI defines the location of these tumors and the degree of infiltration of adjacent structures but is not diagnostic.

On gross examination, fibrosarcomas are lobulated, ill-circumscribed gray-white, firm tumors. Microscopically, they are composed of multiple, pleomorphic spindle cells with focal areas of necrosis. Reticulin staining can demonstrate the collagen network surrounding the cells. These tumors are distinguished from fibrosing mediastinitis by their greater amounts of spindle cell infiltrates containing cytologic evidence of malignancy.

Treatment is by complete surgical excision, although this is rarely possible secondary to advanced infiltration of mediastinal structures. The usefulness of adjuvant radiation or chemotherapy is unknown. While distant metastasis is uncommon, unchecked growth within the mediastinum with early death is the usual course.

13.6.3 Malignant Fibrous Histiocytoma

Although malignant fibrous histiocytoma is the most frequent soft tissue sarcoma of adult life (usually found in the extremities or retroperitoneum), it rarely occurs as a primary mediastinal tumor [77, 85–88]. Most of these tumors in the mediastinum are metastatic.

These tumors have been reported in both the anterior and the posterior mediastinal compartment. In the anterior compartment, they often invade the aorta, and one recent case report describes a primary malignant fibrous histiocytoma associated with a Dacron aortic graft [85–92]. In the eight primary cases that have been reported to date, symptoms have varied greatly depending on the location and size of the tumor. Chest pain, dyspnea, dysphagia, and other complaints have been reported.

Preoperative CT imaging, as well as open incisional biopsy, has been recommended prior to complete excision of these tumors, and a recent report suggests that MRI may be especially helpful in determining the vascular supply and the extent of local invasion [90].

On gross examination, these tumors are poorly circumscribed, multilobulated, infiltrating flesh-colored masses. Histologically, they are composed of pleomorphic spindle cells displayed in a characteristic storiform pattern. They may contain giant and inflammatory cells as well [87]. The spindle cells are immunoreactive to vimentin [77]. Electron microscopy is also useful in establishing the diagnosis [90].

Treatment is based on principles gained from experience with malignant fibrous histiocytoma of the extremities and retroperitoneum. Complete excision with adjuvant radiation and/or chemotherapy is advocated, although clear evidence of a benefit to adjuvant therapy is currently lacking. Unfortunately, local recurrence and distant metastasis are both common.

13.7 Tumors of Muscular Origin

13.7.1 Rhabdomyoma

Rhabdomyoma is a rare lesion of skeletal muscle origin that consists of two types: cardiac and extracardiac. The cardiac type is considered hamartomatous and most often occurs in patients with tuberous sclerosis. Extracardiac types are benign and involve the head and neck areas or the female perineum. Only a single case report exists of an extracardiac mediastinal rhabdomyoma and this was thought to have originated from thymic myoid cells [93]. In this case report, the lesion was discovered at autopsy in an 80-year-old male, and prior to death there were no symptoms present that could be attributed to the tumor. It was located in the anterosuperior mediastinum and on gross examination was an ovular, well-circumscribed mass. The tumor was composed of large polyhedral cells of variable size, with small, eccentric nuclei. These tumors are benign and excision is curative.

13.7.2 Rhabdomyosarcoma

Most cases of rhabdomyosarcoma occur in children and teenagers, and are distinctly unusual after age 21. These tumors of striated muscle origin usually arise in the extremities, head and neck region, or pelvis and are rarely encountered as primary mediastinal tumors [10]. DONALDSON reported that only 2% of 686 of these tumors occurred in the thorax [94]. In their classic paper, PACHTER and LATTES reported only three cases of primary mediastinal rhabdomyosarcoma [6]. KING et al. reported five mediastinal rhabdomyosarcomas in children [4], and CABALLERO et al. recently described two such tumors associated with mediastinal germ cell tumors [95]. Males are affected more than females, with a ratio of 3:2, and, in general, the prognosis is better for children than adults [94]. Symptoms relate to the compression or infiltration of adjacent mediastinal structures, and the tumor is often detected by chest roentograms or CT.

Rhabdomyosarcomas are commonly divided into four histologic types: embryonal, botryoid, alveolar, and pleomorphic. The embryonal type is the most common, accounting for 50% of all cases. The alveolar type accounts for 20%, while the botryoid accounts for approximately 6%. The term "pleomorphic" is no longer commonly used as these tumors are usually classified as malignant fibrous histiocytomas. Only the embryonal and alveolar types have been described in the mediastinum. The alveolar type carries a worse prognosis.

Grossly, these tumors are rubbery and ill circumscribed, with fibrous or myxoid appearing cut surfaces [16]. The embryonal type is composed of small to medium sized round cells with scant eosinophilic cytoplasm, round hyperchromatic nuclei, and occasional rhabdomyoblastic elements. The alveolar type differs in its alveolar appearance, with larger atypical cells lying amidst spaces lined by viable round cells. Histologic diagnosis and classification of rhabdomyosarcoma can be extremely difficult, and often relies on immunohistochemical and electron microscopic evaluation.

The diagnosis of these tumors is usually made by biopsy or examination of the resected specimen. Unfortunately, no definite policy exists regarding the role of surgery. Only a small percentage of patients are candidates for complete excision, and the role of debulking procedures is unknown. Knowledge of local lymph node status is important in directing radiation therapy, and roughly 40% of patients have regional nodal involvement at time of diagnosis [96]. Size of the tumor clearly relates to both degree of local infiltration and nodal involvement. Given these facts, complete excision should be performed if possible.

Radiation and chemotherapy have made significant contributions to the treatment of rhabdomyosarcomas. In 1970, two-thirds of children with this tumor died of their disease. Currently, two-thirds of children with rhabdomyosarcoma survive long-term, and this improvement is clearly secondary to advances in chemotherapy. Doxorubicin, hydrochloride, cyclophosphamide, actinomycin D, and vincristine sulfate are the most common and effective chemotherapeutic agents used [93–98].

Prognosis depends on tumor type, size and presence of metastasis. Distant metastasis is associated with a survival rate of 20%. In the absence of metastasis, survival approaches 80%.

13.7.3 Leiomyoma

Leiomyomas are tumors of smooth muscle origin which, like leiomyosarcomas, are rarely found in the mediastinum and are thought to develop in this location from smooth muscle cells in the media of blood vessels. It is for this reason that some include these tumors in the category of mesenchymal tumors of blood vessel origin. Less than 20 cases of mediastinal leiomyoma have been reported in the world literature [99–101], and most occur in the posterior or middle compartments. These benign tumors are more common in women than men, and have only been reported in adults. Symptoms, if present, relate to compression of adjacent structures. Histologic diagnosis is made either by biopsy or after excision.

Grossly these tumors are well-circumscribed, firm, encapsulated, and exhibit a whorled cut surface on sectioning. They are composed of interlacing bundles of spindle cells set within collagenous stroma. The spindle cells have elongated nuclei with rounded ends.

These lesions are benign and once the correct diagnosis has been established excision is curative.

13.7.4 Leiomyosarcoma

Leiomyosarcomas are malignant tumors that originate from smooth muscle. In the mediastinum, these tumors are usually associated with the media of the great vessels. True primary leiomyosarcomas of the mediastinum that are not associated with tumors of the great vessels are extremely rare, with fewer than five reported in the literature [102–107]. Each of these was a leiomyosarcoma of the superior vena cava. Numerous reports exist, on the other hand, of leiomyosarcomas involving the pulmonary artery and aorta. Most of these cases have involved the pulmonary artery, and most have been intraluminal. These lesions are not considered primary mediastinal tumors.

Grossly, leiomyosarcomas closely resemble leiomyomas. They are gray-white and firm, and the cut surface has a whorled appearance. Microscopically, they are composed of interlacing bundles of large spindle cells, with hyperchromatic nuclei, mitotic figures, and areas of focal necrosis.

The patients with tumors of the superior vena cava presented with symptoms of either chest pain or superior vena caval obstruction. Treatment has consisted of resection of the involved wall of the cava using a partially occluding clamp and replacement with a vein patch or prosthetic graft. More extensive involvement of the cava may require innominate vein (or caval) to atrial bypass of the involved segment with prosthetic graft and en bloc resection of the tumor and superior vena cava. Adequate resection of tumors involving the main pulmonary artery may require prosthetic graft replacement using cardiopulmonary bypass. The role for radiation and chemotherapy is unknown.

13.8 Tumors of Skeletal Tissue Origin

13.8.1 Chondroma, Chondrosarcoma, Osteogenic Sarcoma

There are only a handful of case reports of primary mediastinal tumors with cartilaginous or osteogenic patterns of differentiation, and the extreme rarity of these tumors makes any diagnostic or therapeutic conclusions difficult. Nevertheless, some information regarding the nature of these tumors is available from both the case reports and reports of similar tumors arising elsewhere in the body. For the sake of completeness, each will be discussed briefly.

Only two case reports of extraosseous chondroma exist [108, 109]. The most recent of these reports described a large chondroma arising in the posterior mediastinum of a 19-year-old female [108]. The patient presented with symptoms of dysphagia. Diagnosis of a posterior mediastinal mass was established with use of CT scan, and complete surgical excision resulted in cure. Chondromas of the chest wall are commonly mistaken for mediastinal tumors, particularly in the posterior compartment, where they commonly arise from either the prevertebral bodies or heads of ribs. They are slow-growing, lobulated masses that are impossible to distinguish from chondrosarcomas on clinical grounds [110]. They are composed of lobules of hyaline cartilage and are difficult to distinguish microscopically from low-grade chondrosarcomas. For this reason wide excision is recommended.

Chondrosarcomas are similarly rare primary mediastinal tumors. Only a single case report exists, although numerous other reports describe tumors that are associated with the lung or chest wall [111, 112]. These tumors are clinically and pathologically difficult to distinguish from chondromas. The case report mentioned above described a posterior mediastinal tumor not associated with the chest wall or lung parenchyma. Wide excision of chest wall tumors results in a 97% cure rate. Whether similar outcomes can be expected with adequate excision of primary mediastinal chondrosarcomas is unknown.

Extraosseous osteosarcomas of the mediastinum occur more frequently than the skeletal tumors mentioned above, but they are still extremely rare, with five documented cases in the literature [113, 116]. These lesions have occurred in both the anterior and visceral mediastinal compartments, and some have contained central areas of calcification on CT scan. Microscopically these tumors have an osteoblastic appearance, with malignant-appearing polygonal cells and islands of osteoid. These tumors, when they occur elsewhere in the body, behave aggressively with frequent metastasis to the lungs, bone, and soft tissues. Long-term survival following wide excision is reported as less than 25% [77]. Treatment with wide excision and radiation has been used successfully in patients with primary mediastinal osteosarcoma, but significant information regarding proper treatment is unavailable due to the very limited reported experience.

13.9 Tumors of Pluripotential Mesenchyme

13.9.1 Mesenchymoma (Benign and Malignant)

Mesenchymomas are, by definition, composed of fibrous tissue and two or more unrelated differentiated tissue types (e.g., smooth muscle, cartilage, bone). They are extremely rare in the mediastinum. Several were reported in the large series by PACHTER and LATTES [6], and an additional case of a mediastinal chondrolipoma was reported in 1980 by LIM [117]. Elsewhere in the body these tumors mainly affect adults. Treatment and prognosis depend upon the degree of malignancy.

13.9.2 Synovial Sarcoma

Synovial sarcomas are malignant soft tissue tumors that originate from pluripotential mesenchymal cells which have biphasic epithelial and spindle cell elements. Overall, this is the fourth most common type of soft tissue sarcoma, and it typically occurs in the extremities. Other sites include the head and neck, abdominal wall, and heart. A recent report describes five such tumors that occurred in the mediastinum [118]. In each patient, the tumor arose from the visceral mediastinal compartment. Although some of the tumors were adherent to the pleura or pericardium, they did not arise from these mesothelial lined surfaces. All patients were adult males, and all presented with symptoms of a respiratory nature (cough, dyspnea, and hemoptysis). In each case described, the tumors were large (5–12 cm) and had extensively infiltrated or surrounded adjacent mediastinal structures (aortic arch, left main pulmonary artery, lung).

Microscopically, these tumors are composed of sheets and fascicles of plump spindle cells that show a transition to an epithelioid component. The epithelioid element can either form irregular cellular nests, line intratumoral clefts, or demonstrate glandular or papillary differentiation. The epithelial cells immuno-react with antibodies to keratin, and the spindle cells stain with antibodies to vimentin. These tumors can be very difficult to distinguish from malignant mesotheliomas, thymomas, malignant peripheral nerve sheath tumors, and malignant germ cell tumors (i.e., teratocarcinoma). As with most of the tumors discussed, careful search for a nonmediastinal primary tumor must also be done to rule out metastatic spread to the mediastinum.

Complete excision was not possible in the patients mentioned above. One patient received postoperative radiation therapy, and another received postoperative radiation and chemotherapy. Both of these patients developed pulmonary and chest wall metastasis, and died within 4 years of diagnosis. The patient who received surgery alone died at 10 months of disease, and information regarding the other two patients was unavailable. As in other sites, mediastinal synovial sarcoma is an aggressive tumor that carries an extremely poor prognosis.

13.10 Other Mesenchymal Tumors

13.10.1 Solitary Fibrous Tumor

Solitary fibrous tumor is a neoplasm with multiple names, including benign mesothelioma, submesothelioma, localized fibrous tumor, pleural fibroma, fibrous mesothelioma, localized fibrous mesothelioma, pleural fibroma, and subserosal fibroma. This excessive terminology results from the multiple theories of the origin of this tumor [119–121]. Currently, most believe that this tumor originates from a submesothelial connective tissue cell and not from a mesothelial cell, as previously believed. The evidence for this rests on electron microscopic and immunoreactive studies [122].

While these tumors are uncommon, they occur with greater frequency than many of the tumors discussed in this chapter. In PACHTER and LATTES' series, they represented less than 1% of all mediastinal tumors, but at least 30 cases have been reported in the recent literature [6, 122, 123]. Most of these tumors were located in the anterior mediastinum, although they have been reported in all compartments. Approximately half of the reported tumors were malignant, and nearly all of the patients were male adults. The malignant variety is more likely to produce symptoms, but approximately half of the benign tumors were associated with symptoms in the most recent series [122]. The most common symptoms are cough, chest pain, fever, and dyspnea. Hypoglycemia has also been reported.

On gross examination, these lesions are encapsulated, firm, and lobulated. They vary greatly in size and location. The cut surface is gray with a whorled appearance (Fig. 13.5). Microscopically, these tumors are composed of either a pattern resembling that of the hemangiopericytoma, or a pattern of round to spindle cells amidst dense collagen bundles. Malignant tumors have increased cellularity and mitotic activity, with areas of necrosis and hemorrhage. Immunocytochemistry and electron microscopy are important both in determining degree of malignancy and in differentiating these tumors from mesotheliomas and spindle cell thymomas.

Chest films typically demonstrate a smooth, dense, well-defined mass in the mediastinum (Fig. 13.6). The treatment for solitary fibrous tumors is surgical excision. Complete excision is curative, even for most malignant tumors. Malignant tumors that cannot be completely resected have a high incidence of local recurrence despite radiation and chemotherapy. However, resection of slow-growing, low-grade malignant tumors has been associated with prolonged survival.

13.10.2 Miscellaneous Rare Tumors

Several other rare mesenchymal tumors have been described in the mediastinum. They include meningiomas, chordomas, granular cell tumors, and mediastinal xanthomas. For more information regarding these very unusual tumors, the reader is directed

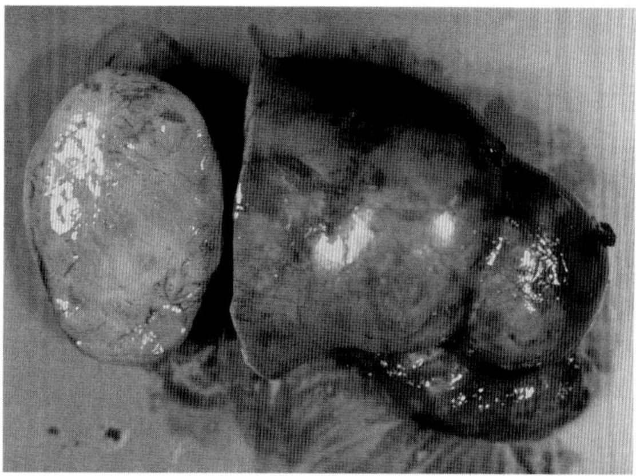

Fig. 13.5. Photograph of a solitary fibrous tumor on cut section

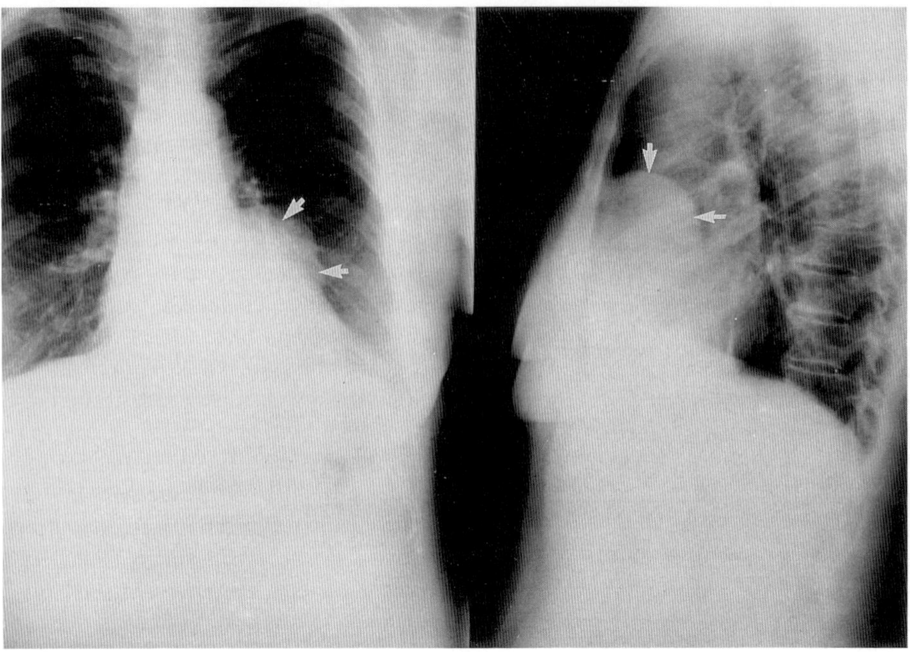

to the isolated reports listed in the references [124–127].

Fig. 13.6. Radiographs of a solitary fibrous tumor (*arrows*) in the anterior mediastinal compartment adjacent to the left heart border

References

1. Wychulis AR, et al. (1971) Surgical treatment of mediastinal tumors: a 40 year experience. J Thorac Cardiovasc Surg 62:379
2. Davis RD Jr, Oldham HN Jr, Sabiston DC Jr (1987) Primary cysts and neoplasms of the mediastinum: recent changes in clinical presentation, methods of diagnosis, management and results. Ann Thorac Surg 44:229
3. Luosto R, et al. (1978) Mediastinal tumors. A follow-up study of 208 patients. Scand J Thorac Cardiovasc Surg 12:253
4. King RM, et al. (1982) Primary mediastinal tumors in children. J Pediatr Surg 17:512
5. Conkle DM, Adkins RB Jr (1972) Primary malignant tumors of the mediastinum. Ann Thorac Surg 14:553
6. Pachter MR, Lattes R (1963) Mesenchymal tumors of the mediastinum (I, II, III). Cancer 16:74
7. Dehner LP (1987) Pediatric surgical pathology, 2nd edn. Williams and Wilkins, New York
8. Blegvad S, et al. (1990) Mediastinal tumors, a report of 129 cases, Scand J Thorac Cardiovasc Surg 24:39
9. Benjamin SP, et al. (1972) Primary tumors of the mediastinum. Chest 62:297
10. Marchecsky AM, Kaneko M (1992) Mesenchymal tumors of the mediastinum. In: Marchecsky AM, Kaneko M (eds) Surgical pathology of the mediastinum, 2nd edn. Raven Press, New York, pp 274–299
11. Brown LR (1986) Intrathoracic lymphangioma. Mayo Clin Proc 61:882
12. Pilla TJ (1982) CT evaluation of cystic lymphangiomas of the mediastinum. Radiology 144:841
13. Fraser P (1989) Diagnosis of diseases of the chest, 3rd edn. Saunders, Philadelphia
14. Perkes EA, et al. (1979) Mediastinal cystic hygromas in infants. Clin Pediatr 18:169
15. Toye R, et al. (1991) Lymphangiohaemangioma of the mediastinum. Br J Radiol 64:62
16. Swanson PE (1991) Soft tissue neoplasms of the mediastinum. Semin Diagn Pathol 8:14–34
17. Baker B, Sherrick DW (1992) Mediastinal lymphangioma. AJR 159:218
18. Pilla TJ, et al. (1982) CT evaluation of cystic lymphangiomas of the mediastinum. Radiology 144:841
19. Brown LR, Aughenbaugh GL (1991) Masses of the anterior mediastinum: CT and MR imaging. AJR 157:1171
20. King DT, Duffy DM, Hirose FM, et al. (1979) Lymphangiosarcoma arising from lymphangioma circumscriptum. Arch Dermatol 115:969
21. Milsom JW, et al. (1985) Chylothorax: an assessment of current surgical management. J Thorac Cardiovasc Surg 89:221
22. Strausser JL, Flye MW (1981) Management of nontraumatic chylothorax. Ann Thorac Surg 31:520
23. Azizkhan RG, et al. (1983) Pleuroperitoneal shunts in management of neonatal chylothorax. J Pediatr Surg 18:842
24. Murphy MC, et al. (1989) Pleuroperitoneal shunts in the management of persistent chylothorax. Ann Thorac Surg 48:195
25. Johnson DW, et al. (1986) Mediastinal lymphangioma and chylothorax: the role of radiotherapy. Ann Thorac Surg 41:325
26. Berberich FR, et al. (1975) Lymphangiomatosis with chylothorax. J Pediatr 87:941

27. Gilsanz V, et al. (1976) Multiple lymphangiomas of the neck, axilla, mediastinum and bones in the adult. Radiology 120: 161

28. Watts MA, Gibbons JA, Aaron BL (1982) Mediastinal and osseous lymphangiomatosis, case report and review. Ann Thorac Surg 34: 324

29. McCarty KS, et al. (1980) Pulmonary lymphangiomyomatosis responsive to progesterone. N Engl J Med 303: 1461

30. Stovin PG (1973) Pulmonary lymphangiomyomatosis syndrome. J Pathol 109: 7

31. Silverstein EF, et al. (1974) Pulmonary lymphangiomyomatosis. AJR 120: 832

32. Vasquez JJ, et al. (1976) Lymphangiomyomatosis. Morphometric study and ultrastructural confirmation of the histogenesis of the lung lesion. Cancer 37: 2321

33. Lack EE, et al. (1986) Pulmonary and extrapulmonary lymphangioleiomyomatosis. Report of a case with bilateral renal angiomyolipomas, multifocal lymphangioleiomyomatosis, and a glial polyp of the endocervix. Am J Surg Pathol 10: 650

34. Cohen AJ, et al. (1987) Mediastinal hemangiomas. Ann Thorac Surg 43: 656

35. Kalicinski ZH, et al. (1982) Hemangioma of the superior caval vein. J Pediatr Surg 17: 178

36. Enzinger FM, Weiss SW (1988) Soft tissue tumors, 2nd edn. Mosby, St. Louis

37. Bedros AA, Munson J, Toomey FE (1980) Hemangioendothelioma presenting as a posterior mediastinal mass in a child. Cancer 46: 801

38. Kelley MJ, Mannes EJ, Ravin CE (1978) Mediastinal masses of vascular origin. A review. J Thorac Cardiovasc Surg 76: 559

39. Kings GLM (1975) Multifocal haemangiomatous malformation: a case report. Thorax 30: 485

40. Rodriguez Paniagua JM, Casillas M, Iglesias A (1988) Mediastinal hemangioma: correspondence. Ann Thorac Surg 45: 583

41. Ginhart TD, Tucker WY, Choy SH (1979) Cavernous hemangioma of the superior mediastinum. Am J Surg Pathol 3: 353

42. Balbaa A, Chesterman JT (1957) Neoplasms of vascular origin in the mediastinum. Br J Surg 188: 36

43. Telander RL, et al. (1984) Prognosis and management of lesions of the trunk in children with Klippel–Trenaunay syndrome. J Pediatr Surg 19: 417

44. Davis JM, Mark GJ, Greene R (1978) Benign blood vascular tumors of the mediastinum. Rad 126: 581

45. Ohmura K, Ishikawa S, Takimoto T, Nishimura T (1991) View from within: radiology in focus. Venous haemangioma of the neck and mediastinum. Path 105: 386

46. Schurawitzhi H, et al. (1991) CT and MRI in benign mediastinal haemangioma. Clin Radiol 43: 91

47. Seline TH, Gross BH, Francis IR (1990) CT and MR imaging of mediastinal hemangiomas. J Comput Assist Tomogr 14: 766

48. Ishii K, et al. (1990) MRI of mediastinal cavernous hemangioma. Pediatr Radiol 20: 556

49. Tourarkissian B, et al. (1990) Mediastinal epithelioid hemangioendothelioma. Ann Thorac Surg 49: 680

50. Weiss SW, Enzinger FM (1982) Epithelioid hemangioendothelioma. A vascular tumor often mistaken for a carcinoma. Cancer 50: 970

51. Yousem SA, Hochholzer L (1987) Unusual thoracic manifestations of epithelioid hemangioendothelioma. Arch Pathol Lab Med 111: 459

52. Abratt RP, et al. (1983) Angiosarcoma of the superior vena cava. Cancer 52: 740

53. Miller MM, et al. (1985) Primary angiosarcoma of the innominate vein: case report with resection and long term survival. J Thorac Cardiovasc Surg 90: 148

54. Galvin IF, et al. (1988) Pericardial hemangiopericytoma as a cause of dysphagia. Ann Thorac Surg 45: 94

55. Kleinhaus S, Ducharme JC (1969) Mediastinal lipoma in children. Surgery 66: 790

56. Politis J, et al. (1979) Intrathoracic lipomas. Report of three cases and review of the literature with emphasis on endobronchial lipoma. J Thorac Cardiovasc Surg 77: 550

57. Mendez G Jr, et al. (1979) Fatty tumors of the thorax demonstrated by CT. AJR 133: 207

58. Shub C, Parkin TW, Lie JT (1979) An unusual mediastinal lipoma simulating cardiomegaly. Mayo Clin Proc 54: 60

59. Lee WJ, Fattal G (1976) Mediastinal lipomatosis in simple obesity. Chest 70: 308

60. Homer MJ, et al. (1978) Mediastinal lipomatosis. CT confirmation of a normal variant. Radiology 128: 657

61. Koerner HJ, Sun KDC (1966) Mediastinal lipomatosis secondary to steroid therapy. AJR 98: 461

62. Shukla LW, Katz JA, Wagner ML (1988) Mediastinal lipomatosis: a complication of high dose steroid therapy in children. Pediatr Radiol 19: 57

63. Tabrisky J, et al. (1974) Benign mediastinal lipoblastomatosis. J Pediatr Surg 9: 399

64. Dudgeon DL, Haller JA Jr (1984) Pediatric lipoblastomatosis. Two unusual cases. Surgery 95: 371

65. Prando A, et al. (1990) Sonographic features of benign lipomatous tumors in children – report of 4 cases. Pediatr Radiol 20: 571

66. Federici S, Cuoghi D, Sciutti R (1992) Benign mediastinal lipoblastoma in a 14 months-old infant. Pediatr Radiol 22: 150

67. Whyte AM, Powell N (1990) Case report: mediastinal lipoblastoma of infancy. Clin Radiol 42: 205

68. Mclean TR, et al. (1989) Mediastinal involvement by myxoid liposarcoma. Ann Thorac Surg 47: 920

69. Prohm P, Winter J, Ulatowski L (1981) Liposarcoma of the mediastinum: case report and review of the literature. Thorac Cardiovasc Surg 29: 119

70. Schweitzer DL, Aguam AS (1977) Primary liposarcoma of the mediastinum. Report of a case and review of the literature. J Thorac Cardiovasc Surg 74: 83

71. Standerfer RJ, Armistead SH, Paneth M (1981) Liposarcoma of the mediastinum. Report of two cases and review of the literature. Thorax 36: 693

72. Dogan R, et al. (1989) Primary mediastinal liposarcoma. A report of a case and review of the literature. Eur J Cardiothorac Surg 3: 367

73. Plukker JTM, et al. (1988) Primary liposarcoma of the mediastinum in a child. J Surg Oncol 37: 257

74. Greiger TA et al. (1988) Mediastinal liposarcoma in a patient infected with the human immunodeficiency virus (letter). Am J Med 84: 366

75. Lacey CJN, Petch MC (1979) Primary liposarcoma of the pericardium. Thorax 34: 120

76. England DM, Hochholzer L, McCarthy MJ (1989) Localized benign and malignant fibrous tumors of the pleura. A clinicopathologic review of 223 cases. Am J Surg Pathol 13: 640

77. Shields TW, Robinson PG (1989) Mesenchymal tumors of the mediastinum. In: Shields TW (ed) Primary mediastinal tumors. Lea & Febiger, Philadelphia, pp 272–288

78. Neinstein LS (1990) Life-threatening desmoid tumor. J Adolesc Health Care 11:453
79. Hill DR, Newman H, Phillips TL (1973) Radiation therapy of desmoid tumors.AJR 117:84
80. Kinzbrunner B, et al. (1983) Remission of rapidly growing desmoid tumors after tamoxifen therapy. Cancer 52:2201
81. Lanari A (1983) Effect of progesterone on desmoid tumors (letter). N Engl J Med 309:1523
82. Barua NR, et al. (1979) Fibrosarcoma of the mediastinum. J Surg Oncol 12:11
83. Baldwin RS (1964) Hypoglycemia associated with fibrosarcoma of the mediastinum. Review of Doege's patient. Ann Surg 160:975
84. Walsh CH, Wright AD, Coore HG (1975) Hypoglycemia associated with a thoracic fibrosarcoma. Clin Endocrinol 4:393
85. Besznyak I, et al. (1985) Malignant fibrous histiocytoma of the mediastinum. Thorac Cardiovasc Surg 33:106
86. Chen W, Chan CW, Mok CK (1982) Malignant fibrous histiocytoma of the mediastinum. Cancer 50:797
87. Mills SA, et al. (1982) Malignant fibrous histiocytoma of the mediastinum and lung. A report of three cases. J Thorac Cardiovasc Surg 84:367
88. Weiss SW, Enzinger FM (1978) Malignant fibrous histiocytoma. An analysis of 200 cases. Cancer 41:2250
89. Paterson HS, et al. (1989) Malignant fibrous histiocytoma associated with a dacron vascular prosthesis. Ann Thorac Surg 47:772
90. Morshuis WJ, et al. (1990) Primary malignant fibrous histiocytoma of the mediastinum. Thorax 45:154
91. Venn GE, et al. (1986) Malignant fibrous histiocytoma in thoracic surgical practice. J Thorac Cardiovasc Surg 91:234
92. Natsuaki M, et al. (1986) Xanthogranulomatous malignant fibrous histiocytoma arising from the posterior mediastinum. Thorax 41:322
93. Miller R, Kurtz S, Powers JM (1978) Mediastinal rhabdomyoma. Cancer 42:1983
94. Donaldson SS (1989) Rhabdomyosarcoma: contemporary status and future directions. Arch Surg 124:1015
95. Caballero C, et al. (1992) Rhabdomyosarcomas developing in association with mediastinal germ cell tumours. Virchows Arch 420:539
96. Pedrick TJ, Donaldson SS, Cox RS (1986) Rhabdomyosarcoma: the Stanford experience using a TMN staging system. J Clin Oncol 3:370
97. Marasco WJ, Hruban RH, Fishman EK (1991) Mediastinal involvement by alveolar rhabdomyosarcoma: evaluation with computerized tomography. South Med J 84:924
98. Maurer HM, et al. (1988) The intergroup rhabdomyosarcoma study-1: a final report. Cancer 61:209
99. Shaffer K, Pugatch RD, Sugarbaker DJL (1990) Primary mediastinal leiomyoma. Ann Thorac Surg 50:301
100. Baumgartner WA, Mark JBD (1980) Esophageal leiomyoma first seen as a mediastinal mass. Arch Surg 115:94
101. Seremetis MG, et al. (1973) Leiomyoma of the esophagus. Ann Thorac Surg 16:308
102. Rasaretnam R, Panabokke RG (1975) Leiomyosarcoma of the mediastinum. Br J Dis Chest 69:63
103. Wick MR, et al. (1982) Primary pulmonary leiomyosarcomas. A light and electron microscopic study. Arch Pathol Lab Med 106:510
104. Henrichs KJ, Wenisch HJC, Hofman W, Klein F (1979) Leiomyosarcoma of the pulmonary artery. A light and electronmicroscopical study. Virchows Arch 383:207
105. Kevorkian J, Cento DP (1973) Leiomyosarcoma of large arteries and veins. Surgery 73:390
106. Davis GL, Bergmann M, O'Kane H (1976) Leiomyosarcoma of the superior vena cava. A first case with resection. J Thorac Cardiovasc Surg 72:408
107. Sunderrajan E, et al. (1984) Leiomyosarcoma in the mediastinum presenting as superior vena cava syndrome. Cancer 53:2553
108. Widdowson DJ, Lewis–Jones HG (1988) A large soft-tissue chondroma arising from the posterior mediastinum. Clin Radiol 39:333
109. Daroczi G (1956) Radikal operiertes Chondrom des hinteren Mediastinums. Zentralbl Chir 81:1245
110. Pairolero PC (1989) Chest wall tumors. In: Shields TW (ed) General thoracic surgery, 3rd edn. Lea & Febiger, Philadelphia, pp 579–588
111. Chelty R (1990) Extraskeletal mesenchymal chondrosarcoma of the mediastinum. Histopathology 17:261
112. Phillips GWL, Choong M (1991) Case report: chondrosarcoma presenting as an anterior mediastinal mass. Clin Radiol 43:63
113. Greenwood SM, Meschter SC (1989) Extraskeletal osteogenic sarcoma of the mediastinum. Arch Pathol Lab Med 113:430
114. Tarr RW, et al. (1988) Primary extraskeletal osteogenic sarcoma of the mediastinum: clinical, pathologic, and radiologic correlation. South Med J 81:1317
115. Ikeda T, et al. (1974) Primary extraskeletal osteogenic sarcoma of the mediastinum. Thorax 29:582
116. Catanese J, et al. (1988) Mediastinal osteosarcoma with extension to the lungs in a patient treated for Hodgkin's disease Cancer 62:2252
117. Lim YC (1980) Mediastinal chondrolipoma. Am J Surg Pathol 3:490
118. Witkin GB, Miettinen M, Rosai J (1989) A biphasic tumor of the mediastinum with features of synovial sarcoma. A report of four cases. Am J Surg Pathol 13:490
119. Goodlad JR, Fletcher CDM (1991) Solitary fibrous tumor arising at unusual sites: analysis of a series. Histopathology 19:515
120. Bortolotti U, et al. (1992) Giant intrapericardial solitary fibrous tumor. Ann Thorac Surg 54:1219
121. Neinstein LS (1990) Life-threatening desmoid tumor. J Adolesc Health Care 11:453
122. Witkin GB, Rosai J (1989) Solitary fibrous tumor of the mediastinum. A report of fifteen cases. Am J Surg Pathol 13:547
123. England DM, Hochholzer L, McCarthy MJ (1989) Localized benign and malignant fibrous tumors of the pleura. A clinicopathologic review of 223 cases. Am J Surg Pathol 13:640
124. Wilson AJ, et al. (1979) Mediastinal meningioma. Am J Surg Pathol 3:557
125. Castellano GC, Johnston HW (1975) Intrathoracic chordoma presenting as a posterior mediastinal tumor. South Med J 68:109
126. Aisner SC, et al. (1988) Bilateral granular cell tumors of the posterior mediastinum. Ann Thorac Surg 46:688
127. Rossi NP, Figueroa PR, Koruss ME (1973) Mediastinal xanthoma with familial hyperlipoproteinemia. Chest 64:144

14 Undifferentiated Carcinoma of the Mediastinum

SHAFIQUE KESHAVJEE and ROBERT J. GINSBERG

CONTENTS

14.1 Introduction

The term "undifferentiated carcinoma (or poorly differentiated carcinoma) of the mediastinum" refers to an epithelial tumor with no histopathologic features allowing precise identification of the site of origin. Approximately 10%–15% of patients with primary mediastinal tumors will be given this diagnosis at the time of biopsy [1]. This diagnostic term encompasses a heterogeneous group of patients, some of whom actually have tumors of well-defined types. A diligent effort should be made to identify those patients so that they may be treated according to standard guidelines for their specific tumor type. Patients with undifferentiated carcinoma of the mediastinum were previously thought to have a uniformly poor prognosis regardless of therapy. However, the group at Vanderbilt University [2] has taken a leading role in demonstrating that these patients can be effectively treated and a few can even be cured with platinum-based chemotherapy.

SHAFIQUE KESHAVJEE, M.D., F.R.C.S. (C), Department of Surgery, Toronto General Hospital, University of Toronto, 200 Elizabeth St., Toronto, Ontario, Canada M5G 117
ROBERT J. GINSBERG, M.D., F.R.C.S. (C), Professor of Surgery, Cornell University Medical College; Chief of Thoracic Service, Department of Surgery, Memorial Sloan-Kettering Cancer Center, 1275 York Avenue, New York, NY 10021, USA

14.2 Classification

Many types of cancer can involve the mediastinum and some frequently have poorly differentiated histology. These include extragonadal germ cell tumors (seminoma or non-seminoma), non-Hodgkin's lymphoma, malignant thymoma, thymic carcinoid, metastatic lung cancer (small cell or non-small cell), undifferentiated soft tissue sarcoma, and other metastatic tumors (Table 14.1). Only when a primary or secondary lung tumor cannot be identified, should the lesion be considered an "undifferentiated carcinoma of the mediastinum."

14.3 Diagnosis

It is essential to use all means available in an attempt to make a specific diagnosis before embarking on therapy because specific treatments exist for many of these tumor types [3] (Table 14.1). The

Table 14.1. Differential diagnosis of undifferentiated tumors of the mediastinum

Extragonadal tumors
  Seminoma
  Nonseminomatous tumor
Lymphoma
  Non-Hodgkin's Lymphoma
Geographic tumor
  Undifferentiated sarcoma
Thymic tumors
  Thymic carcinoma
  Thymic carcinoid
  Malignant thymoma
Metastatic tumors
  Lung
    Small cell
    Non-small cell
  Germ cell
    Seminoma
    Nonseminomatous
  Sarcoma
  Renal cell tumor
Undifferentiated carcinoma

history and physical examination should be used as a guide in the search for a primary site. A chest x-ray and a computed tomographic scan of the chest and abdomen should also be performed on all patients. In most instances these tumors are confined to the anterior (prevascular) mediastinum, but they may involve the superior mediastinum as well. Further radiographic examination should be guided by the patient's signs and symptoms. An exhaustive search for a primary site in the absence of specific signs and symptoms has not been found to be useful [2]. However, detailed examination of the tests (including ultrasound) and pelvic organs (in females) will occasionally reveal a primary germ cell tumor.

In addition to routine laboratory studies all patients should have serum levels of human chorionic gonadotropin and α-fetoprotein measured, as these markers are diagnostic of a malignant germ cell tumor. Fiberoptic bronchoscopy should be performed to search for an occult lung primary tumor, especially in smokers and elderly patients.

Percutaneous fine-needle aspiration or core biopsies do not always provide sufficient tissue for histologic examination and special studies. Thus frequently an incisional biopsy specimen is required. This is usually accomplished by anterior mediastinotomy (Chamberlain procedure) but the CT findings are used as a guide to the optimal approach. Close communication between the surgeon, oncologist, and pathologist is necessary to ensure that an adequate biopsy is taken, that it is handled correctly, and that the appropriate studies are performed (Figs. 14.1–14.3).

When light microscopic examination of an adequately sized biopsy specimen shows a pleomorphic population of large, cohesive malignant cells growing with no definable histologic pattern, further studies should be performed in an effort to obtain a specific diagnosis. These include special stains, electron microscopy, and possibly chromosomal or genetic analysis.

Immunoperoxidase staining techniques can be very useful in the evaluation of poorly differentiated tumors. Positive human chorionic gonadotropin or positive α-fetoprotein stains may suggest a malignant germ cell tumor (even in the absence of elevated serum levels of these markers). Positive common leukocyte antigen and negative keratin stains may suggest a lymphoma. Positive neuron-specific enolase and positive chromogranin stains suggest a neuroendocrine carcinoma.

Positive vimentin and positive desmin stains suggest a poorly differentiated sarcoma. Melanoma is suggested by positive S-100 protein, positive vimentin, and positive desmin stains. Using immunoperoxidase staining techniques, a specific diagnosis was suggested in 20% of these patients [3].

Ultrastructural features discernible by electron microscopic examination can also be useful. This modality is reliable in distinguishing lymphoma from carcinoma and can often definitively diagnose melanoma and poorly differentiated sarcoma.

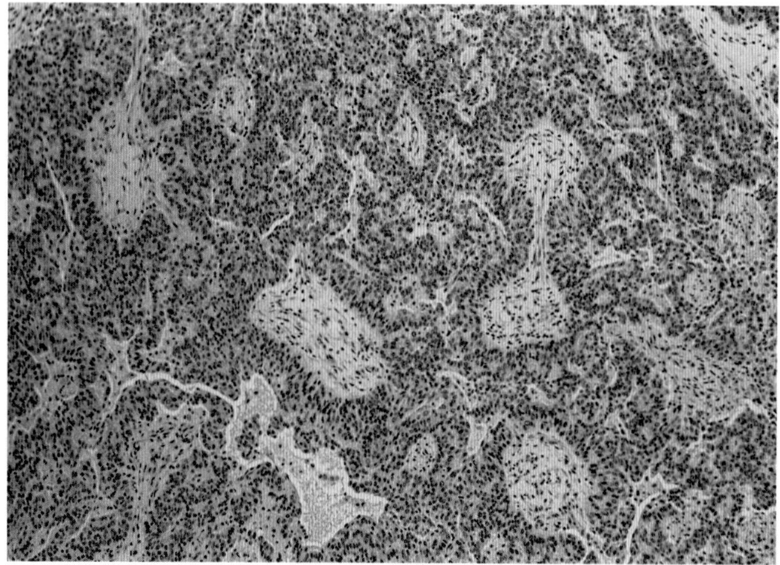

Fig. 14.1. A 45-year-old man presented with chest pain and an anterior mediastinal mass. An anterior mediastinotomy was performed for definitive diagnosis. This photomicrograph demonstrates anastomosing trabeculae and nests of epithelial tumor cells separated by fibrous tissue. (Courtesy of J. Brendan M. Mullen, M.D.) H&E, ×100 (original magnification)

Fig. 14.2. A high-powered view (in the same patient as in Fig. 14.1) shows gland-like spaces lined by cuboidal to columnar cells with vesicular nuclei and prominent nucleoli. There was no evidence of a primary site elsewhere and all tumor markers were negative. (Courtesy of J. Brendan M. Mullen, M.D.) H&E, ×630 (original magnification)

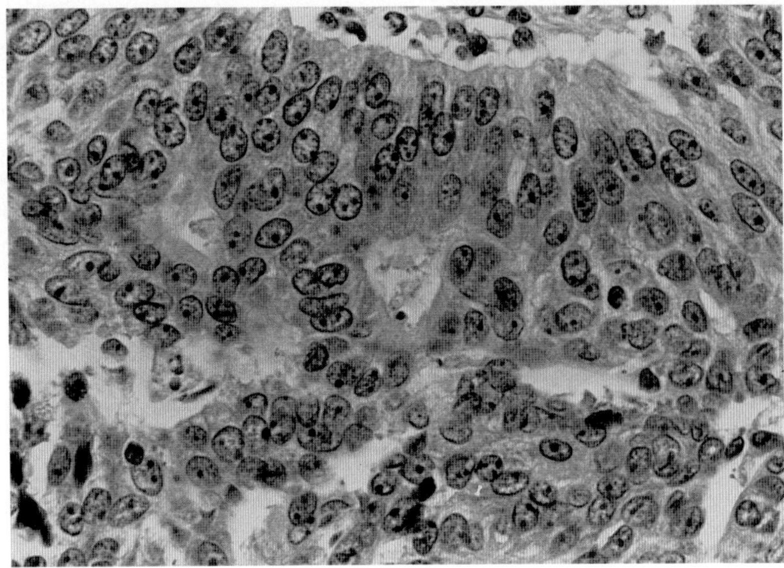

Fig. 14.3. Electron microscopy (in the same patient as in Fig. 14.1) demonstrates intracellular lumen lined by microvilli. Desmosomes are prominent. (Courtesy of J. Brendan M. Mullen, M.D.) ×5700 (original magnification)

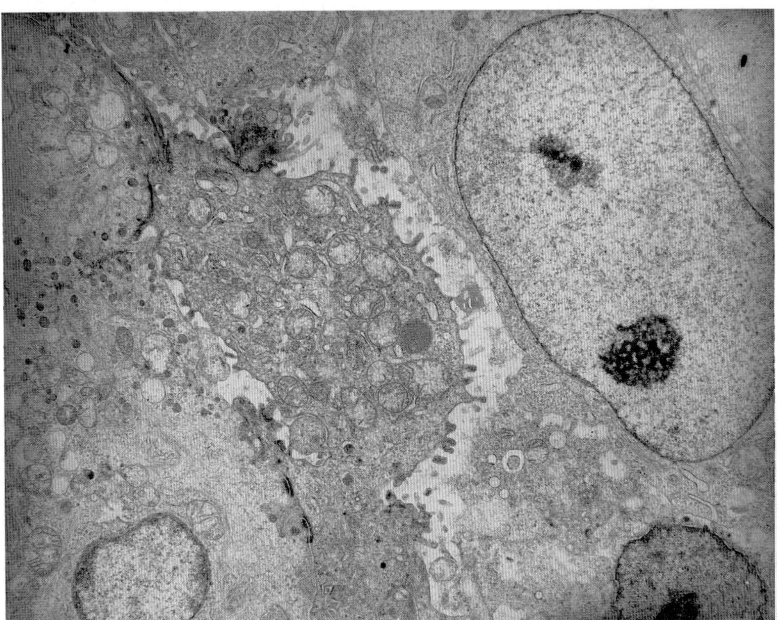

Examination for chromosomal or more specific genetic abnormalities may play a more important role as the genetic basis of malignant disease is elucidated and as genetic markers associated with different cancers are discovered. For example, a large percentage of malignant germ cell tumors have a specific abnormality of the short arm of chromosome 12 [4]. Specific chromosomal abnormalities have also been identified in leukemia, lymphoma, and peripheral neuroepithelioma.

14.4 Treatment (Fig. 14.4)

A few patients with undifferentiated carcinoma with no distinguishing features may have a tumor that is relatively small, is limited to the mediastinum, and does not appear to invade local structures. These patients should be offered total surgical resection. A small number may be cured. The role of adjuvant therapy following complete resection is unknown.

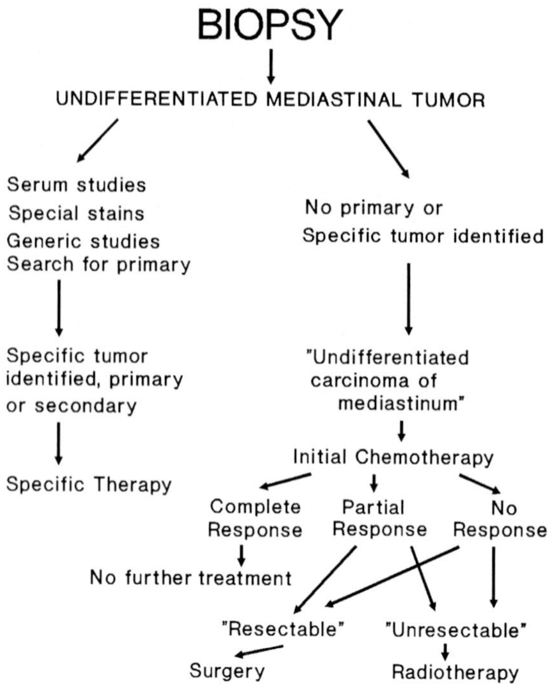

Fig. 14.4. Algorithm for managing undifferentiated tumors of the mediastinum. See text for specific chemotherapy

In some patients, the diagnostic evaluation will define the treatment for certain subsets of patients. Those cases with very high levels of either human chorionic gonadotropin or α-fetoprotein should be treated as malignant nonseminomatous germ cell tumor. Those patients who are found to have an endobronchial lesion and neuroendocrine features by electron microscopy or immunoperoxidase staining should be treated for small cell lung cancer, and those without the neuroendocrine features should be treated for non-small cell lung cancer.

The majority of patients with undifferentiated carcinoma of the mediastinum have bulky unresectable tumors and these require treatment with nonsurgical modalities. Initially, it was thought that some of these patients may represent a subgroup of unrecognized extragonadal germ cell tumors [2]. They were thus empirically treated with cisplatin, vinblastine, and bleomycin (PVeB). The Vanderbilt group has reported a series of more than 200 patients treated with cisplatin-based chemotherapy similar to effective germ cell protocols [2]. Thirty-six percent of the patients had a partial response to therapy and 26% had a complete response. Sixteen percent of the entire group are currently disease-free at a median of 5 years following therapy (1–11 years of follow-up). Actuarial 10-year survival from this study is 16%. Patients with clinical features suggestive of extragonadal germ cell tumors had a higher complete response rate and a higher long-term survival rate (29%) than the group as a whole (Figs. 14.5–14.7).

The results in this study differ from previous reports of patients with carcinoma of unknown

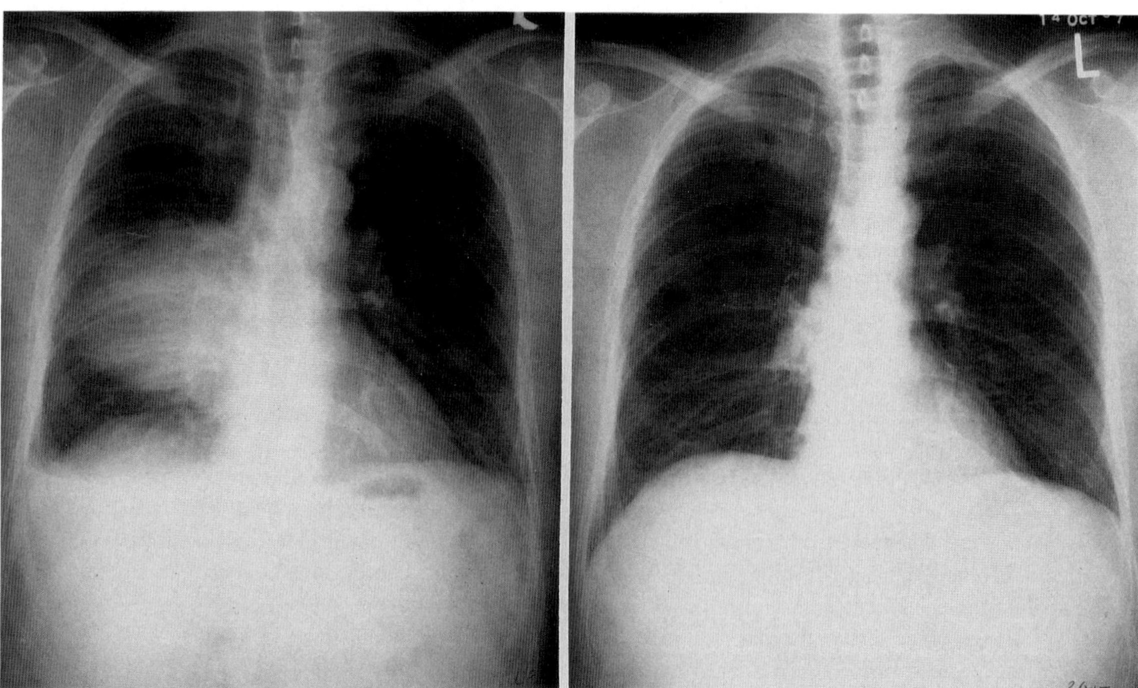

Fig. 14.5. The patient described in Fig. 14.1, showing almost complete resolution of the mass following chemotherapy

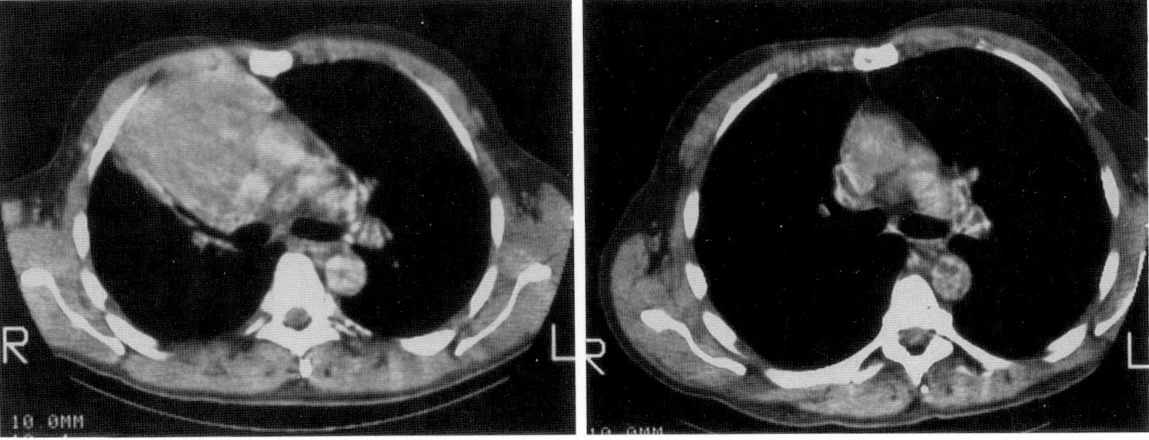

Fig. 14.6. A CT scan of the same patient as in Fig. 14.5. There is no evidence of superior mediastinal disease

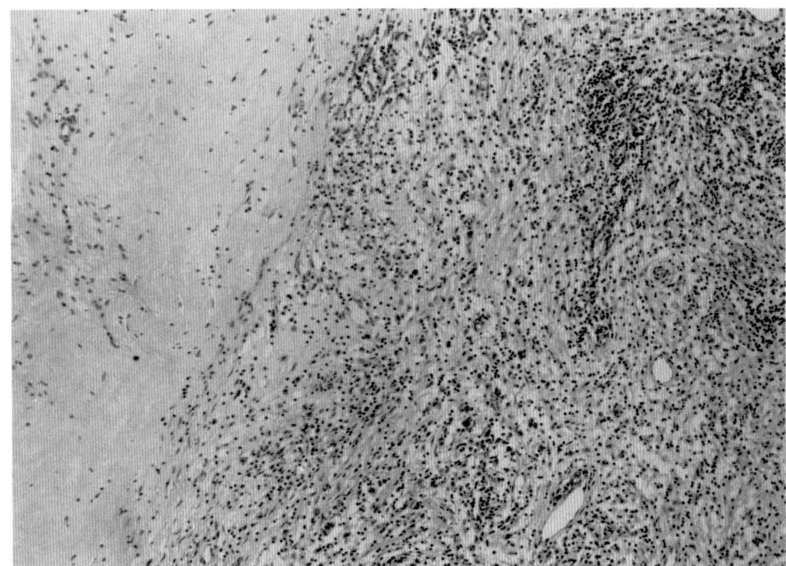

Fig. 14.7. The patient previously described underwent resection of a necrotic mass. This photomicrograph demonstrates necrosis with a chronic inflammatory infiltrate. No active tumor was identified in the specimen. The patient remains well 7 years later. (Courtesy of J. Brendan M. Mullen, M.D.) H&E, ×100 (original magnification)

primary site, in which no long-term disease-free survivors have been reported with any non-cisplatin-containing chemotherapy regimen [2].

Although some of the highly responsive patients likely have germ cell tumors that are marker-negative and unidentifiable using currently available pathology methods [2], it is felt that the responsive tumors represent a heterogeneous group. In the Vanderbilt experience, some of the tumors responsive to cisplatin-based chemotherapy were ultimately found to be non-Hodgkin's lymphoma, poorly differentiated neuroendocrine tumors, melanoma, and malignant thymoma. This unusual group may be a unique subset of chemotherapy-sensitive tumors and some may even represent a previously undefined tumor type. Alternatively, it is speculated that some may represent highly undifferentiated, and therefore chemotherapy-sensitive, epithelial tumors from occult primary sites that are usually much less responsive to systemic therapy.

In those tumors responding to chemotherapy, if only a partial response is identified (versus a complete response) it has been our practice to attempt a total excision of the residual tumor. In many cases, a fibrotic mass, devoid of tumor, will be resected. On occasion this continued treatment, even with residual disease present, will be curative. If this appears impossible because of local organ invasion, radiotherapy of the residual mass may be worthwhile. In those tumors unresponsive to chemotherapy, radiotherapy may be of value but rarely cures.

14.5 Conclusion

The diagnosis of "undifferentiated carcinoma" of the mediastinum refers to a heterogeneous group of mediastinal tumors. Experience gained over the past decade has shown that this is not a hopeless group of patients. They should no longer be treated with palliative radiotherapy or symptomatic treatment alone on the assumption that they are incurable. Optimal clinical and pathologic examination can establish a more specific diagnosis with specific therapy in some of these patients. Furthermore, a few of those who are still classified as "undifferentiated carcinoma" after detailed clinical and pathologic examination can be cured with intensive platinum-based chemotherapy and thus should be offered a trial of this treatment. The current first-line treatment recommended by the Vanderbilt group is the combination of cisplatin, etoposide, and bleomycin. This regimen is felt to be at least as active as cisplatin, vinblastine, and bleomycin, but less toxic. Responses are expected to be rapid in this group; thus therapy should be discontinued if no response is observed after one or two courses.

References

1. Adkins RB, Maples MD, Hainsworth JD (1984) Primary malignant mediastinal tumors. Ann Thorac Surg 38: 648–659
2. Hainsworth JD, Johnson DH, Greco FA (1992) Cisplatin based combination chemotherapy in the treatment of poorly differentiated carcinoma and poorly differentiated adenocarcinoma of unknown primary site: results of a 12 year experience. J Clin Oncol 10: 912–922
3. Hainsworth JD, Greco FA (1991) Poorly differentiated carcinoma of the mediastinum. In: Shields TW (ed) Mediastinal surgery. Lea and Febiger, Philadelphia, pp 225–227
4. Motzer RJ, Rodriguez E, Reuter VE, et al. (1991) Genetic analysis as aid in diagnosis for patients with midline carcinoma of uncertain histologies. J Natl Cancer Inst 83: 341–346

15 The Role of Three-Dimensional Conformal Radiotherapy in the Treatment of Mediastinal Tumors

MACK ROACH III and SRINIVASAN VIJAYAKUMAR

CONTENTS

15.1 Introduction

Although considerable clinical experience has been accumulated in applying three-dimensional (3-D) technology to the treatment of prostatic carcinoma, the potential value of this technology in the management of thoracic neoplasms has only recently been recognized [1–10]. A variety of factors have contributed to this "lag" in the routine use of 3-D based technology for the management of thoracic neoplasms. First, the routine implementation of 3-D conformal radiotherapy (3-DCRT) has been hampered by the lack of widespread availability of FDA-approved 3-D software. The labor-intensive nature of 3-DCRT and the failure of many radiation oncologists to recognize the shortcomings of standard treatment techniques have also contributed to the slow diffusion of 3-D technology. Most investigators who have access to 3-D based treatment planning are convinced that the potential benefits associated with its routine use will ultimately result in its widespread adoption. To test the hypothesis that this technology will result in improved local control and possibly survival, phase I/II dose

MACK ROACH III, M.D., Associate Professor, Department of Radiation Oncology, University of California, School of Medicine, 505 Parnassus Avenue, San Francisco, CA 94143-0226, USA
SRINIVASAN VIJAYAKUMAR, M.B.,B.S., D.M.R.T., Associate Professor, Department of Radiation and Cellular Oncology, University of Chicago/Pritzker School of Medicine, Chicago, Illinois, USA

escalation studies sponsored by the Radiation Therapy Oncology Group (RTOG) are underway. In this review we discuss how this "tool" may allow us to improve the treatment of mediastinal tumors.

15.2 "Beam's Eye View" and "Room's Eye View"

Several of the potential benefits associated with the use of 3-DCRT are listed in Table 15.1. Despite the emphasis placed by some investigators on the potential for dose escalation, accurate targeting may be the most important of these benefits [6, 7]. The ability to generate treatment plans using a so-called beam's eye view (BEV) makes this accurate targeting possible [7, 12]. The BEV is similar to viewing a target through the sight of a high-powered rifle. In the case of BEV-associated tumor targeting, all treatment angles are theoretically possible. For instance, VIJAYAKUMAR et al. compared 3-D and conventional radiation therapy planning in lung cancer in 21 patients [13, 14]. They found that there were significant deficiencies with conventional planning in terms of target volume coverage. The angles and field sizes generated using 3-D treatment planning were different in more than 70% of the patients, when all the CT information available was used. Optimized oblique angles that would probably not have been chosen (because of overlapping shadows and the associated uncertainty of precise

Table 15.1. Potential benefits of 3-D based conformal radiotherapy

1. Improved accuracy of tumor targeting
2. Nonconventional beam angles to allow sparing of normal tissues
3. Greater dose delivery while keeping the dose to surrounding structures within tolerance
4. Uniform definitions of tumor volumes, clinical target volumes, and dose prescription
5. Ability to define the partial dose/volume tolerances of normal tissues more accurately

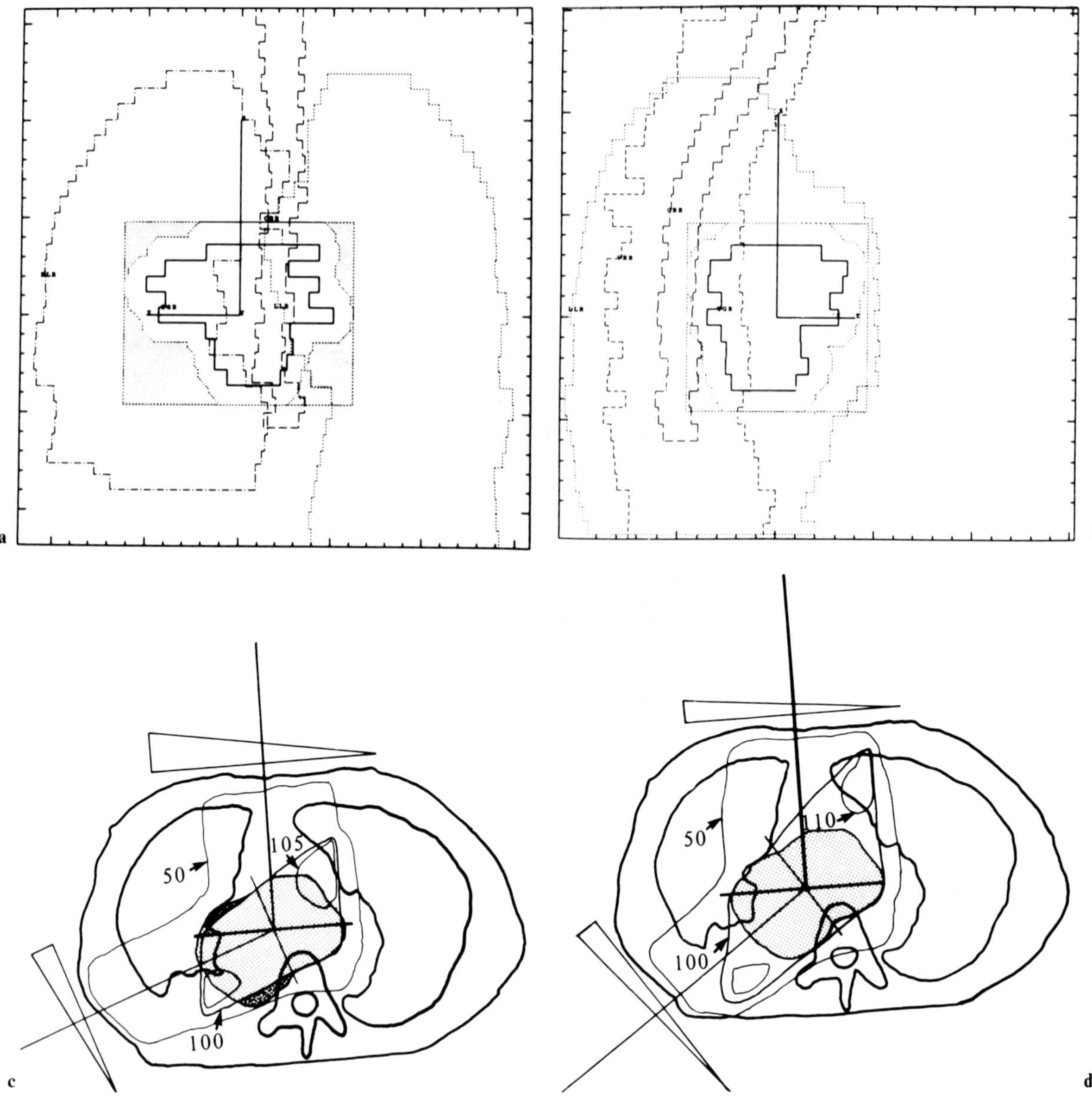

tumor location) can be readily identified. Transparent overlays can be generated by the computer using margins specified by the radiation oncologist. These transparencies can be placed directly on simulation films and the blocks designed. Whether accurate target definition is the most important benefit or not, it is clear that none of the other benefits are likely to be realized without accurate target definition.

In addition to the BEV, 3-D technology allows treatment displays using the "room-view" or "rooms eye view" (REV) [15]. Using this display format, the relationship of multiple beams to the patient can be observed simultaneously. This allows planners to take into account the impact of the chosen treatment

Fig. 15.1. a A BEV for an anterior field and **b** a BEV for a lateral field. Both were generated using a 3-D CT reconstruction. **c** Set of AP and right posterior oblique beams designed without use of the BEV and attempting to cover a mediastinal mass. Note that a small portion of the tumor is outside the 100% isodose line. **d** Set of AP and right posterior oblique beams generated using the BEV. Note that all of the tumor is inside the 100% isodose line. [7]

technique on other structures which may be out of the central plane of treatment but may be receiving incidental irradiation. The use of the REV may also facilitate setting the patient up for treatment. By generating sagittal REVs demonstrating where on the patient's surface beams enter, the therapist can get a general idea of how the setup should look once done properly.

Figures 15.1a and 15.1b demonstrate AP and lateral BEVs for a patient with a mediastinal mass. Figures 15.1c and 15.1d compare a set of beams designed with (15.1d) and without (15.1c) use of the BEV. Note how the blocks conform to the shape of this mass so that surrounding normal tissues are selectively excluded using an AP beam and a lateral beam. Without use of the BEV, as shown in Fig. 15.1c, part of the tumor is missed in the oblique. The presence of overlapping shadows resulting from mediastinal structures makes it difficult to accurately define the tumor and the spinal cord. Note that using the BEV, as shown in Fig. 15.1d, the optimal angle and blocks can be easily defined.

15.3 Dose Volume Histograms

Another major characteristic of 3-D based technology is the ability to generate dose volume histograms (DVHs) to compare plans. DVHs provide a graphic representation of the relationship between doses of radiation delivered and the volume of tumor and normal tissues irradiated. Using this planning tool, multiple treatment plans can be compared and the one giving the best coverage of the tumor and maximum sparing of critical normal tissues can be selected. For example, Figs. 15.2 and 15.3 represent DVHs for the lungs and spinal cord, respectively, for a patient treated with three different plans. Note that plan 2, using anterior posterior as well as a right anterior oblique and a left posterior oblique (ANT/POST/RAO/LPO), results in a higher dose to the right lung than either plan 1 or plan 3 (Fig. 15.2). In contrast to the relative advantages associated with using plan 3 for sparing the lungs, more than 25% of the spinal cord would receive more than 80% of the dose using this plan (Fig. 15.3). Plan 1, using an anterior superior and inferior obliques and a posterior (ASO/AIO/POST), results in a relatively low dose to both the spinal cord and the right lung. This kind of analysis can be used to compare various treatment techniques to improve the therapeutic ratio of radiation dose to tumor and surrounding normal tissues.

Studies based on patients with prostatic cancer have demonstrated that the use of 3-D based planning has resulted in a reduction in acute toxicity as predicted from DVH-based analysis [3, 4].

Although studies based on patients with thoracic neoplasms have demonstrated better coverage of tumor volumes, the impact on acute and long-term toxicity is only beginning to be defined [6–10]. Recent studies conducted at the University of Michigan suggest that this may be the case for lung cancers as well. These investigators demonstrated that using 3-DCRT, patients with lung cancers can be treated to higher than conventional doses without unacceptable toxicity [11].

The similarity of anatomy between different patients with prostatic cancer has allowed a number of investigators to adopt standard treatment techniques based on a fixed number of coplanar or noncoplanar beams and beam angles, obviating the need for the development of unique treatment plans for each patient [1–5]. Several of the reasons why the use of 3-DCRT in the management of thoracic neoplasms has lingered behind its application in the treatment of prostatic cancer are shown in Table 15.2.

There is much greater anatomic variation in patients with thoracic neoplasms than in patients with prostatic cancer. The optimal treatment technique for treating a thoracic primary is likely to vary dramatically depending on the size, location, and risk of spread to regional nodes [16]. The normal tissues in close proximity to the prostate (the bladder, rectum, and femoral heads) generally have a higher radiation tolerance than the normal tissues adjacent to a thoracic neoplasm (the spinal cord, heart, and lungs), but the doses required to control tumors in both sites appear to be similar. The use of 3-D based radiotherapy for thoracic neoplasms has also been hampered by the need for a relatively large final boost volume and the uncertainties associated with predicting the risk and location of regional metastasis [12, 16].

15.4 The Value of Nonconventional Beam Angles

Some of the potential advantages associated with use of 3-DCRT to treat mediastinal tumors are sum-

Table 15.2. Factors limiting the benefits of 3-DCRT in the treatment of thoracic tumors

1. Wide variation in location of lesions
2. Relatively low tolerance of adjacent normal tissues
3. The type of morbidity associated with excessive irradiation of adjacent normal tissues
4. Greater uncertainity in predicting the location and risk of spread resulting in larger fields

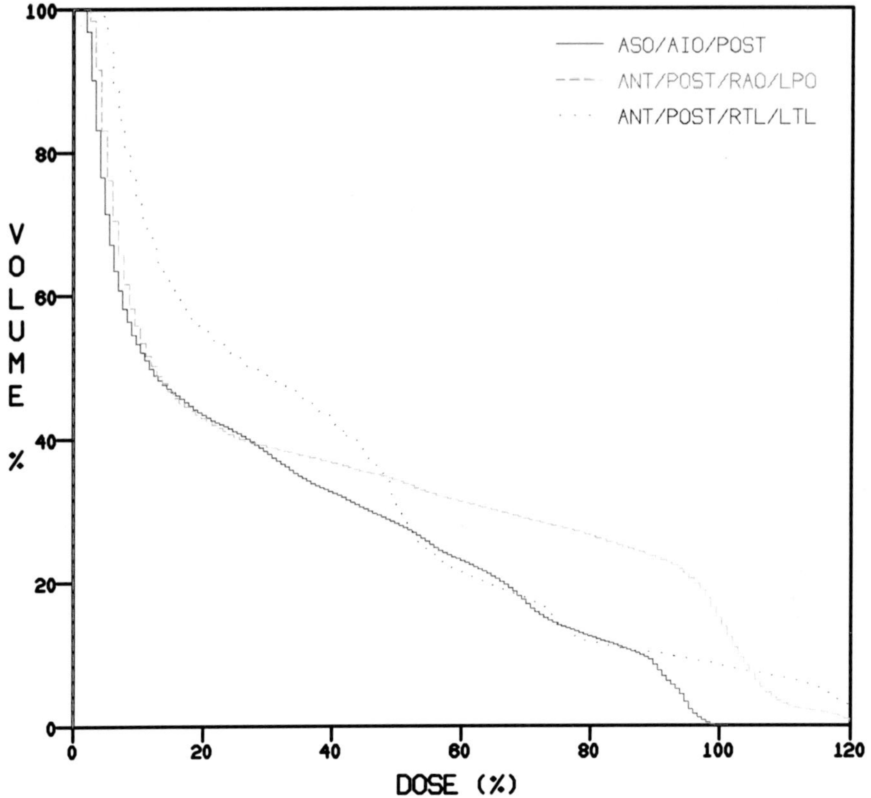

15.2

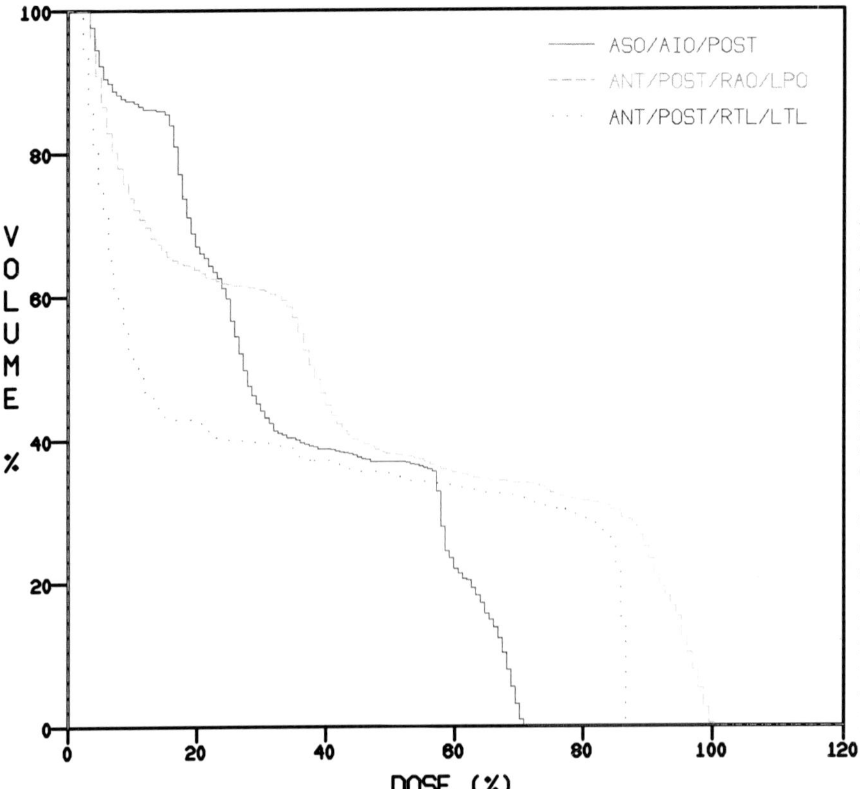

Fig. 15.2, 15.3. DVHs for the lung (Fig. 15.2) and spinal cord (Fig. 15.3) for a patient treated with three different plans. Plan 2, using AP-PA and a right anterior oblique and a left posterior oblique (ANT/POST/RAO/LPO), results in a higher dose to [greater than 25% of] the right lung than either plan 1 or plan 3 (Fig. 15.2). Plans 2 and 3 result in more than 25% of the spinal cord receiving more than 80% of the dose (Fig. 15.3). Plan 1, using an anterior superior and inferior obliques and a posterior (ASO/AIO/POST), results in a relatively low dose to both the spinal cord and the right lung

15.3

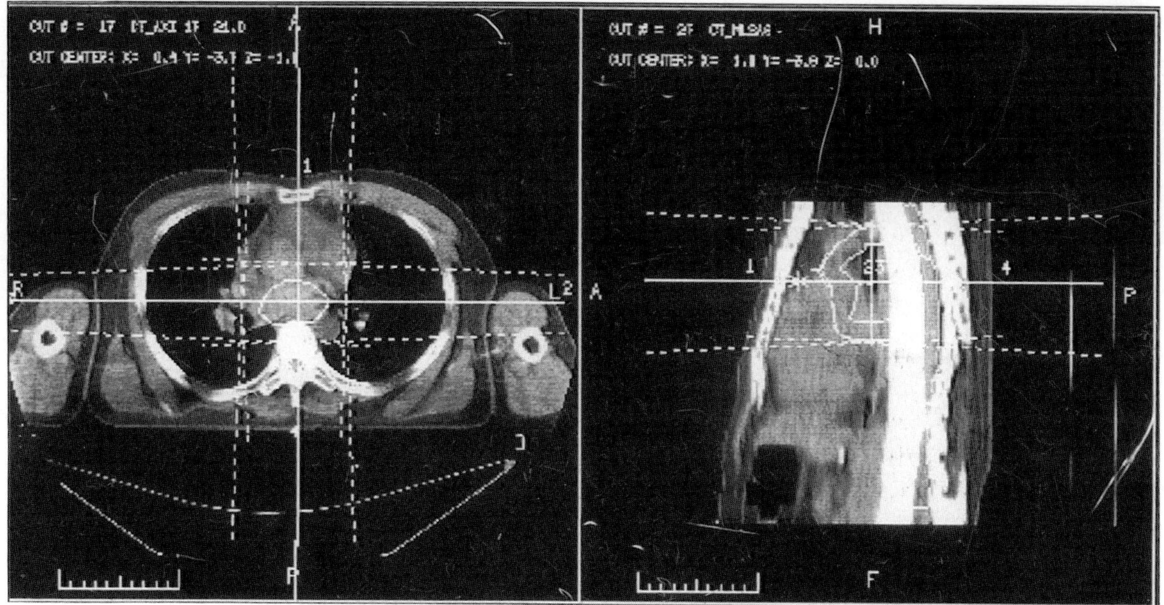

a b

Table 15.3. Advantages of 3-DCRT in the treatment of mediastinal tumors

---

1. Less variation in the location of lesions allows the use of a standardized technique
2. The close proximity of dose-limiting normal tissues magnifies the benefits of 3-DCRT
3. Because of the central location much of the lung can be spared during dose escalation
4. Lower risk of extramediastinal spread?

Fig. 15.4a, b. A conventional technique (AP-PA and laterals) that is frequently used to treat mediastinal tumors. Note that the laterals shown in **b** result in a relatively large volume of normal lung being irradiated

marized in Table 15.3. If involvement by tumor is limited to the mediastinum, it may be possible to develop an optimized "standard treatment plan," without having to "start from scratch" [17, 18]. Figure 15.4 illustrates a conventional technique (AP-PA and laterals) that is frequently used to treat mediastinal tumors. Figure 15.5 illustrates how 3-DCRT can be used to provide tumor coverage and at the same time minimize the dose to surrounding lung. Note that by using two beams in the sagittal plane a greater volume of normal lung can be spared, compared with use of the standard technique. Preliminary work completed at the University of California San Francisco suggests that this type of technique is particularly useful for tumors arising from the posterior mediastinum [19].

While tumors requiring higher doses of radiation such as non-small cell lung cancer, esophageal cancers, and sarcomas would appear to be the most obvious to benefit from the higher doses allowed with 3-DCRT, radiosensitive tumors (germ cell tumors, lymphomas) are also likely to benefit from

the improved tumor localization and the sparing of surrounding normal tissues.

15.5 Miscellaneous Benefits of Three-Dimensional Conformal Radiotherapy

Another benefit which is likely to result from the widespread use of 3-DCRT is the adoption of more uniform language and criteria for specifying target volumes [20]. VALLEY and MIRIMANOFF compared the treatment techniques for a typical lung case in ten Swiss radiation oncology centers. In addition to differences in the treatment techniques used, there were significant variations in the definitions of the target volume, prescription procedures, total dose, and dose per fraction [20]. The availability of CT-based images that can be reconstructed in three dimensions will allow these volumes to be compared rigorously, to be sent electronically, and to be stored for future comparisons. These capabilities will facilitate the development of more uniform definitions for target and treatment volumes [21].

The consequences of these improvements in the reproducibility of CT-based target definitions are likely to be further enhanced by the use of functional measures that can be used to quantitate the

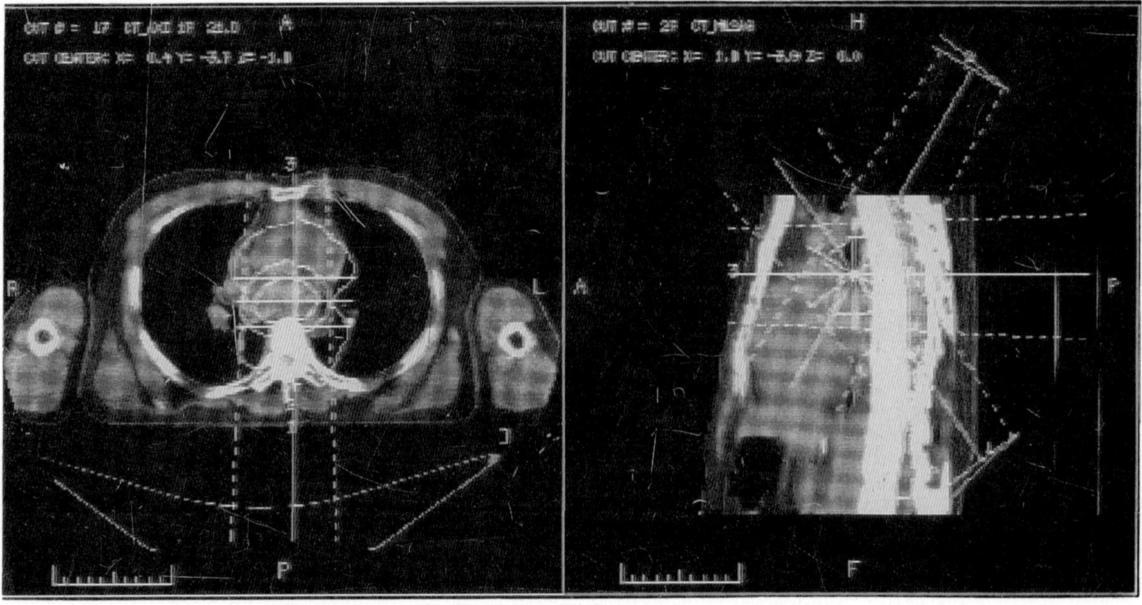

Fig. 15.5a, b. Example of a plan using two beams in the sagittal plane to reduce the volume of normal lung irradiated, compared with use of the standard technique. Note that the sagittal beam shown in **b** spares more of the normal lung because smaller points of the normal lung are in the entrance and exit portions of this beam (compare Fig. 15.4b with 15.5b)

physiologic consequences of thoracic irradiation. For example, MARKS et al. used 3-D single-photon emission computed tomography lung perfusion scans to define quantitatively regions of dysfunction which would not otherwise have been recognized [22]. They frequently found marked variations in regional function that were not necessarily immediately adjacent to the tumor volume. They found these pretreatment scans to be useful in designing portals to minimize irradiation of functioning lung. Hopefully by respecting the tolerances of normal tissues and by appropriate use of systemic agents we will be able to improve the cure rate [23, 24]. Combining the 3-D treatment planning technology with 3-D based functional imaging should allow the optimal treatment technique to be defined and the maximum amount of lung to be spared. The reduction in lung volume

irradiated should in turn reduce pulmonary toxicity [23].

15.6 Conclusions

The literature reviewed and the examples shown demonstrate how 3-D based treatment planning technology can allow a higher dose of radiation to be delivered to the mediastinum while minimizing the

Table 15.4. Selected series using 3-DCRT for treatment of thoracic neoplasms

Authors, year[a]	Tumor type	Authors' conclusions
EMAMI et al. 1991 [6]	Lung cancer	Potential for dose optimization, improved tumor coverage, and sparing of normal tissues
VIJAYAKUMAR et al. 1991 [7]	Lung cancer	Beam's eye views facilitate customized treatment planning customized treatment planning
LANGER et al. 1991 [8]	Lung cancer	Restriction of target dose inhomogeneity during 3-D planning has a critical impact
HODAPP et al. 1991 [9]	Lung cancer	Value of CT simulation based 3-D planning
ARMSTRONG et al. 1993 [10]	Lung cancer	Superior dose delivery at reduced risk to surrounding normal tissues
HAZUKA et al. 1993 [11]	Lung cancer	Feasibility of using 3-DCRT to treat patients to high doses (median = 67.6 Gy) without unacceptable toxicity
PURDY et al. 1993 [15]	Not specific	Value of using "room-view" displays and real time interactivity
ROACH et al. 1994 [19]	Mediastinal tumors	Tumor location has a important impact on the usefulness of 3-DCRT

[a] Reference number shown in brackets

dose to surrounding normal tissues. Table 15.4 summarizes some of the conclusions reached by various authors. The phase I/II dose escalation trial being conducted by the RTOG should provide us with a basis for assessing the potential impact of this technology on toxicity and local control and eventually form the basis for a phase III trial to allow us to answer the question, "Do higher doses result in better local control and longer survival?"

Acknowledgements. The authors would like to acknowledge the contibutions of the technical staff, including Barby Pickett MS, who generated some of the example plans shown. Special thanks to Deborah and Sarah Roach for their editorial support.

References

1. Ten Haken RK, Perez-Tamayo C, Tesser RJ, McShan DL, Fraass BA, Lichter AS (1989) Boost treatment of the prostate using shaped, fixed fields. Int J Radiat Oncol Biol Phys 16: 193–200
2. Roach M, Pickett B, Phillips TL (1993) An analysis of the advantages as well as the physical and clinical limitations of three-dimensionally (3-D) based coplanar conformal external beam irradiation (XRT) in the treatment of localized prostate cancer. In: Minet P (ed) Three-dimensional treatment planning. European Association of Radiology 5th Workshop on 3-D Treatment Planning, Liege, Belgium. pp 149–161
3. Soffen EM, Hanks GE, Hunt MA, Epstein BE (1992) Conformal static field radiation treatment of early prostate cancer versus non-conformal techniques: a reduction in acute morbidity. Int J Radiat Oncol Biol Phys 24: 485–488
4. Vijayakumar S, Awan A, Karrison T, et al. (1993) Acute toxicity during external-beam radiotherapy for localized prostate cancer: comparison of different techniques. Int J Radiat Oncol Biol Phys 25: 359–371
5. Sandler H, McLaughlin PW, Haken RT, Addison H, Forman J, Lichter A (1993) 3D conformal radiotherapy for the treatment of prostate cancer: low risk of chronic rectal morbidity observed in a large series of patients. Proceedings of the 35th ASTRO Meeting. Int J Radiat Oncol Biol Phys 27 (Suppl 1): 135
6. Emani B, Purdy JA, Manolis J., et al. (1991) three-dimensional treatment planning for lung cancer. Int J Radiat Oncol Biol Phys 21: 217–227
7. Vijayakumar S, Myrianthopoulos LC, Rosenberg I, Halpern HJ, Low N, Chen GTY (1991) Optimization of radical radiotherapy with beam's eye view techniques for non-small cell lung cancer. Int J Radiat Oncol Biol Phys 21: 779–788
8. Langer M, Kijewski P, Brown R, Ha C (1991) The effect on minimum tumor dose of restricting target-dose inhomogeneity in optimized three-dimensional treatment of lung cancer. Radiother Oncol 21: 245–256
9. Hodapp N, Boesecke R, Schlegel W, Bruggmoster G, Wannemacher M (1991) Three-dimensional treatment planning for conformal therapy of a bronchial carcinoma. Radiother Oncol 20: 245–249
10. Armstrong JG, Burman C, Leibel S, Fontenla D, Kutcher G, Zelefsky M, Fuks Z (1993) Three-dimensional conformal radiation therapy may improve the therapeutic ratio of high dose radiation therapy for lung cancer. Int J Radiat Oncol Biol Phys 26: 685–689
11. Hazuka MB, Turrisi AT, Lutz ST, et al. (1993) Results of high-dose thoracic irradiation incorporating beam's eye view display in non-small cell lung cancer: a retrospective multivariate analysis. Int J Radiat Oncol Biol Phys 27: 273–284
12. Perez CA, Stanley K, Grundy G, et al. (1982) Impact of irradiation technique and tumor extent in tumor control and survival of patients with unresectable non-oat cell carcinoma of the lung. Cancer 50: 1091–1099
13. Vijayakumar S, Myrianthopoulos LC, Rosenberg I, Halpern HJ, Low N, Chen GTY (1991) Optimization of radical radiotherapy with beam's eye view techniques for non-small cell lung cancer. Int J Radiat Oncol Biol Phys 21: 779–788
14. Vijayakumar S, Low N, Chen GTY, et al. (1991) Beam's eye view-based photon radiotherapy, I. Int J Radiat Oncol Biol Phys 21: 1575–1586
15. Purdy JA, Harms WB, Matthews JW, et al. (1993) Advances in 3-dimensional radiation treatment planning systems: room-view display with real time interactivity. Int J Radiat Oncol Biol Phys 27: 933–944
16. Minet P, Constant ML, Biquet JF, Lemaire (1993) Probability of lymph node invasion in lung cancer: a tool to delineate the target volume. In: Minet P (ed) Three-dimensional treatment planning, European Association of Radiology, Liege, Belgium, pp 57–68
17. Kukolowicz P, Michalski W, Bulski W (1993) Threshold integral dose optimization criterion. In: Minet P(ed) Three-dimensional treatment planning, European Association of Radiology, Liege, Belgium, pp 199–206
18. Langer M, Brown R, Kijewski P, Ha C (1993) The reliability of optimization under dose-volume limits. Int J Radiat Oncol Biol Phys 26: 529–538
19. Roach M, Pickett B, Kuerth S, Yuo H-S, Phillips TL (1994) The impact of tumor location on the benefits of 3-D based high-dose conformal thoracic irradiation. International Congress for Lung Cancer Meeting, June 22–26, 1994, Athens, Greece
20. Valley J, Mirimanoff R (1993) Comparison of treatment techniques for lung cancer. Radiother Oncol 28: 168–173
21. Emami B, Lyman J, et al. (1991) Tolerance of normal tissue to therapeutic irradiation. Int J Radiat Oncol Biol Phys 21: 109–122
22. Marks LB, Spencer DP, Bentel GC, et al. (1993) The utility of SPECT lung perfusion scans in minimizing and assessing the physiologic consequences of thoracic irradiation. Int J Radiat Oncol Biol Phys 26: 659–668
23. Byhardt RW, Martin L, Pajak TF, Shin KH, Emami B, Cox JD (1993) The influence of field size and other treatment factors on pulmonary toxicity following hyperfractionated irradiation for inoperable non-small cell lung cancer (NSCLC)-analysis of a radiation therapy oncology group (RTOG) protocol. Int J Radiat Oncol Biol Phys 27: 537–544
24. Arriagada R, LeChevalier T, Quoix E, et al. (1991) Effect of chemotherapy on locally advanced non-small cell lung carcinoma: a randomized study of 353 patients. Int J Radiat Oncol Biol Phys 20: 1183–1190

Subject Index

List of Contributors

Mark S. Allen, MD
Assistant Professor of Surgery
Section of General Thoracic Surgery
Mayo Clinic
200 First Street S.W.
Rochester, MN 55905
USA

Jacob D. Bitran, MD
Clinical Professor of Medicine
Division of Hematology/Oncology
Department of Medicine
University of Chicago
Lutheran General Hospital
1875 Dempster Street, # 405
Park Ridge, IL 60068-1129
USA

Leigh Delbridge, MD, FRACS
Professor of Surgery
Endocrine Surgical Unit,
Royal North Shore Hospital
Sydney
Australia

Brent De Vries, DO
Fellow, Division of Cardiology
Department of Medicine
Lutheran General Hospital
1875 Dempster Street, # 405
Park Ridge, IL 60068-1129
USA

L. Penfield Faber, MD
Professor of Surgery
Rush Medical School
Chief of General Thoracic Section
Senior Attending, Department of Cardiovascular
and Thoracic Surgery
Rush-Presbyterian St. Luke's Medical Center
1725 W. Harrison Street
Chicago, IL 60612
USA

Robert J. Ginsberg, MD, FRCS (C)
Professor of Surgery
Cornell University Medical Center
Chief of Thoracic Service
Department of Surgery
Memorial Sloan-Kettering Cancer Center
1275 York Avenue
New York, NY 10021
USA

Thomas W. Griffin, MD
Professor and Chairman
Department of Radiation Oncology, RC-08
University of Washington
1959 NE Pacific Street
Seattle, WA 98195
USA

Richard F. Heitmiller, MD
Assistant Professor of Surgery
Division of General Thoracic Surgery
Osler 624
Johns Hopkins Hospital
600 N. Wolfe Street
Baltimore, MD 21205
USA

Shafique Keshavjee, MD, FRCS (C)
Department of Surgery
Toronto General Hospital
University of Toronto
200 Elizabeth Street
Toronto, Ontario MSG 117

Wui-Jin Koh, MD
Associate Professor
Department of Radiation Oncology, RC-08
University of Washington
1959 NE Pacific Street
Seattle, WA 98195
USA

JOHANNE LeBLANC, MD
Clinical Assistant Professor
University of Washington
Department of Radiology
Group Health Cooperative of Puget Sound
215 15th-Ave E
Seattle, WA 98102
USA

ROBERT B. LEE, MD
Assistant Professor of Surgery (Cardiothoracic)
The Emory Clinic
1365 Clifton Rd. NE
Atlanta, GA 30322
USA

PATRICK J. LOEHRER, Sr., MD
Professor of Medicine
Section Hematology and Oncology
Indiana University School of Medicine
101 W. 10th Street
Indianapolis, IN 46202-2879
USA

WILLIAM J. MARASCO, MD
Russell H. Morgan Department of Radiology
and Radiological Science
Johns Hopkins Medical Institution
600 N. Wolfe Street
Baltimore, MD 21205
USA

DOUGLAS J. MATHISEN, MD
Associate Professor of Surgery
Harvard Medical School
Associate Visiting Surgeon
General Thoracic Surgical Services
Massachusetts General Hospital
Boston, MA 02114
USA

JOSEPH I. MILLER, Jr., MD
Professor of Surgery
Division of Thoracic Surgery
The Emory Clinic
25 Prescott Street, Suite 3417
Atlanta, GA 30308
USA

STEPHEN H. PETERSDORF, MD
Assistant Professor
Division of Medical Oncology, RC-08
University of Washington
1959 NE Pacific Street
Seattle, WA 98195
USA

THOMAS S. REEVE, FRACS, FACS
Professor Emeritus
University of Sydney
Royal North Shore Hospital
Sydney, Australia

MACK ROACH III, MD
Associate Professor
Department of Radiation Oncology
University of California
School of Medicine
505 Parnassus Avenue
San Francisco, CA 94143-0226
USA

JONATHAN SOMERS, MD
Assistant Professor of Surgery
Rush Medical School
Assistant Attending in Cardiovascular
and Thoracic Surgery
Rush-Presbyterian St. Luke's Medical Center
1725 W. Harrison Street
Chicago, IL 60612
USA

CHARLES R. THOMAS, JR., MD
Fellow, Department of Radiation Oncology, RC-08
Former Assistant Professor, Division of Oncology
Department of Medicine
University of Washington
1959 NE Pacific Street
Seattle, WA 98195
USA

SRINIVASAN VIJAYAKUMAR, MBBS, DMRT
Associate Professor
Department of Radiation and Cellular Oncology
University of Chicago/Pritzker School of Medicine
29th Ellis Avenue
Chicago, IL 60616
USA

JOHN C. WAIN, MD
Assistant Professor of Surgery
Harvard Medical School
Director, Lung Transplant Program
General Thoracic Surgical Services
Massachusetts General Hospital
Boston, MA 02114
USA

EARLE W. WILKINS, JR. MD
Clinical Professor of Surgery (em)
Harvard Medical School
Massachusetts General Hospital
32 Fruit Street
Boston, MA 02114
USA

DOUGLAS E. WOOD, MD
Section of General Thoracic Surgery
Division of Cardiothoracic Surgery
Department of Surgery, SA-25
University of Washington
Seattle, WA 98195
USA

CAMERON D. WRIGHT, MD
Assistant Professor of Surgery
Harvard Medical School
Assistant Surgeon
General Thoracic Surgical Services
Warren 1212
Massachusetts General Hospital
Boston, MA 02114
USA